The Process of Psychothe

This book is dedicated to all those who recognize themselves in these pages and travelled part of the road

Senior commissioning editor: Mary Seager
Development editor: Caroline Savage
Production controller: Chris Jarvis
Desk editor: Claire Hutchins
Cover designer: Fred Rose

The Process of Psychotherapy
A Journey of Discovery

Phil Barker and Bobbie Kerr

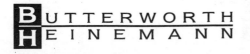
BUTTERWORTH
HEINEMANN

OXFORD AUCKLAND BOSTON JOHANNESBURG MELBOURNE NEW DELHI

Butterworth-Heinemann
Linacre House, Jordan Hill, Oxford OX2 8DP
225 Wildwood Avenue, Woburn, MA 01801-2041
A division of Reed Educational and Professional Publishing Ltd

℞ A member of the Reed Elsevier plc group

First published 2001

British Library Cataloguing in Publication Data
A catalogue record for this book is available from the British Library

Library of Congress Cataloguing in Publication Data
A catalogue record for this book is available from the Library of Congress

ISBN 0 7506 5178 4

Typeset by Avocet Typeset, Brill, Aylesbury Bucks
Printed and bound in Great Britain by Clays Ltd, St Ives plc

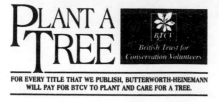

Contents

Authors' note		vi
Prologue		vii
Preface		xiii
1	The search for healing counsel	1
2	Life as drama	19
3	Exploration	35
4	Words – the bridge between two worlds	50
5	Mutuality	67
6	The promotion of growth and development	89
7	The leap of faith	112
8	The glory of discovery	135
9	The road to nowhere	149
Index		171

Authors' note

What follows is an account of the experience of psychotherapy – or at least *some* experiences – for both patient and therapist. We focus mainly on how we made sense of the process, rather than emphasizing what exactly was the focus of therapy, or how the therapy 'worked'. In that sense, this may prove to be an unconventional account of therapy.

The therapeutic story involves four characters; the patient (BK) and two of the three therapists who first attempted to address her problems – the counsellor and the analyst. The fourth therapist (PJB) is referred to throughout as 'the therapist'.

In order to distinguish the experiences of the patient and the therapist this text has been indented, with the patient's text appearing in *italic*.

Prologue

A view from the future

Dear Phil,

I have a feeling I don't know where I am going with this project, only that I am making my way somewhere. This may be significant, since it was my experience of therapy. Making a start was so difficult, then and now. But always I am grateful that I did start and saw it through to the end. As someone a lot smarter than you once said, 'the journey of a thousand miles begins with one step'.

Much of what has stayed with me and was helpful then is deceptively simple. The wise sentences that were passed on and have stayed to spur me or comfort me still were as likely to have been plagiarized from a previous patient as from the ancient philosophers and medical mandarins.

The bottom line was always, is it helpful? A banal platitude was fine if it worked. A tried and tested method would be abandoned if it got me nowhere. At least that was my helpful experience with you – it was different with other therapists.

All I can discuss is my individual experience of therapy – what was helpful and what was not; even what might have been more helpful if tackled a little differently. So what, the reader might well ask. Well, that individual experience spanned a small handful of different therapists with very different approaches. At the time I would rant and rage against them, but at this remove I hope to make a more dispassionate assessment of their methods and vested interests.

As I begin this book, now two years after formally being discharged from therapy, I wonder how difficult it will be to think myself back into the person I was at various stages along the road. How easy will it be to be able to retell the story, when necessary, as it seemed to me then? The person I was then seems so far removed from the person I am now. Yet it is important to be able to return to the starting point and trace the passage before we can take any useful overview from the distance.

I am assisted in this task by letters and notebooks from the period of

*therapy. These did not begin as a formal assignment; indeed one thera-
pist actively discouraged the writing, taking the view that our therapeutic work would not succeed unless I could 'face the demons eyeball to
eyeball'. For myself, I always found writing cathartic. The 'demons'
always troubled me inconveniently, often in the wee small hours, and
rarely during the scheduled hour of therapy. Writing was simply a way I
could sort out my own thoughts when I was alone. Addressing the therapist via the written word was a way of gaining access when he was probably tucked up in bed, dreaming pleasant dreams.*

*Mercifully, I persisted with the writing and eventually found my way to
your door. Far from rejecting my chosen medium, you were encouraging
– and even interested – in these detailed reports of what was happening
in my head at any given moment. Mostly it was straight reportage, with
no immediate intention of distilling the significance of the experiences
noted. I would feel driven to write things down, performing in the process
some kind of exorcism of the demons. The exorcism seems to have been
temporary at first. Many of the themes recur again and again in the writings of the time. Although I didn't realize it then, this work helped me
move away from reliance on a therapist to explore a more independent
life. It was writing, alone, that helped me see a situation or problem and
eventually find the way forward.*

*As I realized I was entering the final sessions of therapy with you, I
drew up a list of outstanding matters I still wanted to deal with. I felt I
had been privileged to have the opportunity to work with someone who
could teach me so much. I was aware such an opportunity was unlikely
to come again, and I wanted to be sure I had exploited it to the full. But
on my last day of therapy, as I scanned my notes of 'outstanding matters',
I moved on down the list, leaving many of the entries unmentioned. I realized that I wasn't going to sort everything out in that meeting – or any
number of others. Most of the items on the list were issues that I, and I
alone, could address.*

*Now I know that the work is finished when I realize the work will never
be finished. There is no 'cure'. There will always be dilemmas, tragedies
and problems. That is what being alive is all about. The work has suc-
ceeded when the one being helped realizes that she no longer needs to
rely on the helper. She is the source of her own solutions. It still happens
occasionally that I lose confidence in myself, in my ability to judge
others. Something happens that shows I have misjudged someone, given
too much trust or not enough. I will be troubled, and on rare occasions I
might feel I'm back at square one, but I can always lay hands on a few
basic therapeutic tools that were given to me. I always seem to get the job
done when I am patient with myself and persist.*

*This then must be the way forward with this new challenge. As I face
this blank screen I have ideas of what I want to say, but wonder if I can
marshal them into a useful form. The starting process, at least, involves
a mirroring of therapy. I wonder if I can make a start. Then I feel frus-*

trated and rage at myself. Finally I just have to take a deep breath and plunge in, hoping it will work but not being quite sure.

Yours

Bobbie

Dear Bobbie

It is good to hear that you are still 'on the road'. As I look back on our work together, I am tempted to pick out only the therapeutic 'high spots'. This is the Achilles' heel of all therapists; the tendency to assume that we *do* anything of any great value, far less that we *know* anything of any lasting worth. Having spent the 'golden hour' with the patient, as you say, the therapist then toddles off to dream pleasant dreams, leaving the patient to continue wrestling with her demons. I would be lying if I said that I never took you home with me in my thoughts. My discipline is such, however, that I found little difficulty in letting you 'float back' to the consulting room, thereby returning me to my slumbers. Perhaps some of that discipline has rubbed off on you and you too have learned how to use the emotional 'left luggage'.

Which reminds me of that apocryphal tale of the two monks who encountered an attractive young woman by the banks of a river. The older of the two monks offered to carry her across and, having deposited her safely on the other side, bid her farewell and continued on his way. After journeying some miles in silence, the older monk stopped to ask his partner what was on his mind. The young monk was incensed. Had he forgotten that their order was sworn to celibacy? What was he thinking of carrying such an attractive woman across the river? The old monk paused: 'Oh, her,' he replied. 'Yes, I left her miles back down the road, but I see that *you* are still carrying her!'

On re-reading your letters and reports, I suspect that learning how to leave your footsteps behind you was one of the invisible tasks you have accomplished. True, like me, you often turn your head and retrace those footprints, frequently acutely aware of what it felt like to be in those shoes at that time. But then you return your attention to here and now and, perhaps more importantly, to the road ahead. *How* you did that is the simple yet remarkably complex story of this book; one that may hold out hope to lay readers who can relate directly to your experiences, and to therapists and would-be therapists who also need infusions of hope. How you achieved the ability to 'live your life' will be the medium for this book.

I intend no disrespect when I say that you have a gift for describing the ordinary nature of everyday life. *Keeping going, climbing, striving, building, creating, discovering and noticing* – these are the ingredients of living. *Arriving* should be the last thing on our minds, for by then it will all be over – quite literally. Life is a protracted process of *becoming*. That kind of a *living* must surely be the core of the 'good life', which so many seek but so few appear to find. Therapy is usually about discovering how a difficult life can, somehow, be made a better life. It is reasonable therefore that learning how to live life should occupy the heartland of the therapeutic endeavour.

Wasn't it Benjamin Franklin who said something to the effect that a long life may not be good enough, but a good life was always long enough? I am sure that he would have endorsed Swift's blessing: 'May you live all the days of your life'.

I am left thinking that if my words encouraged you to do anything, it was nothing more profound than that. But then again there may be nothing more profound than that!

Kierkegaard observed that life 'can only be understood *backwards*'. Much therapy operates on this premise. However, there is a danger that we neglect the second half of Kierkegaard's dictum that, although it may be understood backwards, life '*must be lived forwards*'. I recall once saying in an interview that all I did as a therapist was to help people to live their lives forward. I don't think the interviewer was impressed. It sounds a lot less exciting than exorcizing demons or otherwise mending broken minds.

I have long felt that I do not belong to any 'school' of therapy, and this will be reinforced greatly here in this book, where my 'pick and mix' approach to therapy could be called eclectic by the generous of spirit. However, many psychotherapists might be unhappy that I should even care to describe what I did with you as therapy. Still, I believe that 'psychotherapy', when it does achieve some healing of the mind, must involve a reinventing of oneself. If the patient remains the same, then nothing of any note has happened. I have never been in therapy in the proper sense, but have, I believe, spent much of my adult life inventing and reinventing myself. Given that experience, I appreciate how the process of personal change, at whatever level and depth, is a task that only *you* can realize – a task in which the therapist is a mere onlooker or confidante. Successful therapy results, in my view, in the recognition that one's golden achievement in life is the constant remaking of yourself so that, at last, you know how to live. Once you own that knowledge, then you can begin to make sense of the past. Perhaps you even begin to grasp Emerson's logic when he said that 'most of the shadows of this life are caused by standing in our own sunshine'.

Given that words are such an important part of your life and have played such a key part in our therapeutic dialogue, it is only fitting that the record of your therapy should conclude with these reflections: I always received them in the spirit of a 'therapeutic gift', and I continue to receive them in that spirit. When the only therapy that I might be allowed to practise has become the one-way street of emotional correction that I have, all too often, read about, I shall turn to gardening or some other enlightening pursuit – for clearly I shall need such enlightenment. Albert Einstein once said that he reminded himself a hundred times a day that his inner and outer life depended on the labours of other people, living and dead. Einstein knew that he needed to exert himself in order to give in anything like the measure he had received, and was still receiving. Wise words indeed. These words could be crafted into a plaque to adorn any therapist's office. I shall return, no doubt over and over again, to the gifts that I have received from the many patients with whom I have been privileged to be associated. It will be interesting to see what I can make of the gifts I have received from you.

I sense that much of what lies before you involves courage. It may well be appropriate that you are uncertain of the path, far less the destination. We dare to be wise about the everyday business of living. Those who postpone the hour of living are akin to the traveller waiting for the river to run out before they risk the crossing. There are so many variants of the therapeutic message – from my grandmother's 'there is no time like the present' to the modern Nike's 'Just do it!' All these encouragements require is the courage to enact them, but the message remains an enduringly wise one.

Before I close, I thought that I should say something about my professional part in this whole process. A professor is, as the saying goes, 'someone who talks in someone else's sleep'. But I would add that the professor is (often) someone whose job is to tell students how to solve the problems of life, which he (usually) has tried to avoid by becoming a professor. And so it might well be with therapists, although many will take issue with this judgement. They might go as far as to say 'speak for yourself', which of course I do. Like you I have little idea where this will lead me, but I can feel, as my Irish forefathers would say, the road rising up to meet my every step. I have little understanding of who I am, and even less of what lies before me. Such ignorance is what makes life interesting, if not meaningful. My bags are packed and the journey promises to be likewise.

Yours

Phil

Preface

This book has been a long time in the making. Why that should have been the case isn't entirely clear. We both set to the task with great gusto within two years of the completion of the therapy. The time seemed to be ripe for another set of reflections, albeit a very different set from those that had characterized the original therapist–patient[1] relationship. A protracted hiatus developed, which at one point seemed to threaten the whole project. The evidence suggests strongly that it was the therapist who was dragging his feet, or perhaps even 'resisting' the whole process of reflecting and writing. The usual battle-lines of the life-narrative were drawn out: competing demands from work and life in general, procrastination and promises, promises and yet more promises. The 'truth', if such a near-mythical beast remains of interest to the disaffected reader, probably revolved around the changes that had been taking place, largely anonymously and certainly invisibly, in the relationship between the people who once had been defined as 'therapist' and 'patient'. Although we shall not enter into any further interpretation here, the reader needs to be aware that the text, as it emerges in this book, is a multilevel phenomenon, and certainly derives from at least three stages in the lives of the persons formerly known as the 'patient' and 'therapist'. The process of reflecting on our records and our emotional memories of the experience of therapy engendered yet more records and, more importantly, new thoughts and feelings. It would be altogether too simplistic to say that these new emotions – and the thinking and reflecting with which they cohabit – were *born* of the older reflections. Instead, the way we both feel (similarly and differently) about the experience of therapy is, in part, a revelation (in the proper sense of the word); laying bare some of the dimensions of the experience which appear to have escaped us the first time around. This was a dynamic process. We hope the reader will engage with this

---

[1]For almost forty years people have been attempting to de-stigmatize the consumers of psychiatry or psychotherapy by calling them first clients, and then, more recently, users or consumers. We choose to employ the politically incorrect term 'patient' since, as its Latin root betrays, it appropriately acknowledges the 'suffering' associated with the experience of mental distress, even when that suffering is temporary. In its other common meaning, it denotes what is required of the person as (s)he waits for change to manifest itself or for various mental health professionals – whether therapists or otherwise – to do something useful or meaningful.

dynamism.

If this book is about any *one* thing, it involves the drawing of a map of the territory of therapy as we experienced it. Perhaps the map that emerges will help to provide a perspective for those who have never ventured onto that dark terrain. It may even provide those who have traversed this often hidden region of the human experience with an alternative depiction of some of the more obvious features of this landscape. We would, however warn both these kinds of readers that appearances are often deceptive. Although an accurate and hopefully meaningful account follows, the names are not to be confused with the things they represent. *The map, certainly, is not the territory* (Korzybski, 1933). What we shall speak of here as 'therapy' involves, in many senses, a tour of the patient's private world, and what this tour came to mean for the therapist. We hope to show how that tour can become a journey. We shall try to use our words intentionally, as we do here, where we acknowledge that the life as a 'tour' can often involve a sense of 'going round', often repeating experiences; whereas the 'journey' (Fr. *Jour*) is focused on a new experience that each day may bring. In our view, that *jour*-ney is synonymous with discovery. Perhaps that discovery might even involve the birth of a new experience, each day – *jour-née*. We have laboured our explanation of (or excuses for) the birth of the book merely to emphasize the endlessness of the life journey and the discoveries that it involves about ourselves and others. Although, for us, the book is finished, what it represents – the process of becoming, of both patient and therapist – will never be finished.

Life is an anecdotal medium, and we shall employ anecdotes, new and old, in our efforts to reveal the life lived within this therapeutic relationship. We shall explore how the patient journeyed to the therapist's door; what struggles had already been witnessed; and what kind of shape she was in at the start and how that shape changed. It goes without saying, however, that there never was any journey, any struggle or any shape, as such. These are the dimensions of the metaphorical world of both patient and therapist. In our view, that world of metaphor is more real (in an experiential sense) than reality – or at least the consensual reality to which most of us refer when the Big R is mentioned. Hopefully this will not be read as some trite existential philosophy. This is the truth of human experience – that rarely can we express anything of any value (or truth) concerning our experience that is not couched in metaphor, which essentially is the appropriate but incorrect wrong use of language. As Aristotle noted, metaphor consists in giving a name to a thing that belongs to something else (McKeown, 1941). That great critic of psychiatry Thomas Szasz noted, sagaciously, that the sickness, the dis-ease, the distress, indeed the *illness* that is called 'mental illness', is no more than metaphor – albeit a powerful one (Szasz, 1987). If we fail to appreciate the metaphorical standing of mental distress, we risk failing to grasp its significance – that human experience is so close to ineffability that we need to give it a name that, in truth, belongs to another. The puzzling nature of such metaphorical understandings threads its way through this text. They express not only the patient's difficulties in elucidating her experience, but also those of the therapist, who is doubly handicapped by the popular myth that, given his position and standing, he is *bound* to know something worth knowing.

Much of what we shall discuss, from the perspectives of both patient and therapist, will involve metaphors; expressions that represent the essence of the experience more fully than would any naturalistic description, even if we could find such descriptions. In that sense we expect to discuss 'reality' very rarely, but shall devote more attention to the representation of experience; its essential meaning. We shall be focused, also, more on the significance of the discussion for the therapist. Patients do not, by and large, read books about the experience of psychotherapy, if only because there are few accounts written of such experiences, especially by both patient and therapist. It is also clear that patients are invariably too busy wrestling with their own direct experiences to be too bothered with the experiences of others. In that sense, patients are already learning important lessons. We hope that people who are, have been, or fear that they might become psychotherapy 'patients' will read this book so that they might have an experience against which to match their own. They might also feel less ignorant of what can go on within the therapeutic relationship, as well as of what might conceivably go wrong.

This book might also be of interest to therapists, and indeed all who are even remotely interested in what therapists do, perhaps because they harbour a fancy to join this group. Through our conjoint reflections, we hope an understanding will emerge of some of what needs to be done in the name of the therapeutic exchange.

Our reflections are predicated on three simple questions:

1. Despite our recognition that this is a business largely focused on 'hearing', we shall consider 'how should therapists *look upon*[2] therapy? Perhaps this contradiction reflects our appreciation of the importance of the 'territory'.
2. Despite the obvious fact that it is the patient who is laying her emotional security on the line, to what extent is the therapist really *committed* for that *golden hour*?
3. Given the balance between hearing a version of an age-old tale and encountering something wholly beyond his ken, how does the therapist get in the *right frame of mind* to become effective?

It goes without saying that the focus of the patient's narrative involves weaving together, almost seamlessly, something of her past, much of her present, and what she can grasp of her future. Whether or not this is made explicit at the outset, therapy can hardly begin – and certainly does not continue – without the prerequisite of this human tapestry. Although it is rarely acknowledged, the therapist needs to weave a smaller version of himself in the process of the exchange. Even in that most extreme form of therapy, psychoanalysis, where the therapist infrequently retires behind the 'blank screen', allowing the patient to 'project' whatever images of herself are, at that moment, important, the patient will weave an image of the therapist, whether he likes it or not (Barker, 1999).

What we do not address is also important; sins of omission invariably are. We

---

[2]At the risk of patronizing the reader, we emphasize again the metaphors deployed here in our overview of the book.

offer little insight into the mechanics of therapeutic technique, or the details of the structure of the therapy. Although these are alluded to, our emphasis is upon 'what happened' – experientially. Readers who wish to read more about the kind of therapy models invoked in our therapeutic exchange will find some directed reading in the references, but no more. (For an introduction to the various therapy models, see Barker, 1999). Neither do we devote much detail to the 'outcome' of therapy, popularly addressed today by highly abstract references to changes in numerical scores on various rating scales or questionnaires. The evaluation of progress was entirely qualitative – or, we might say simply, *human.* Any judgement as to whether progress was being made or not was made conjointly, in conversation. Certainly it was not the therapist's task to determine progress, since he was not actually taking the journey but merely following the patient on some short sections of her overall therapeutic encounter. The focus was, unashamedly, on what the patient 'made' of therapy throughout the experience, and what this meant to her in terms of progress. As the narrative will reveal, this was no smooth progression, but was characteristically erratic. Life is invariably erratic, and the life of therapy appears to be no different. Suffice it to say that someone who was sufficiently distressed to be deemed in need of residential psychiatric care and treatment at the beginning of therapy recovered (according to her own standards) sufficiently to write this account of her experience. Perhaps that represents a pudding imbued with some meaningful proof.

We have tried, here, to model a different kind of revelation about therapy. We hope that it does not smack too much of self-congratulation, for, on reflection, perhaps there was much that others might consider had gone awry. That is the whole point of this meta-reflection. However, this was a successful coming together of two strangers, for the avowed purpose of benefiting one person directly and benefiting the other much more covertly. Indeed, that might well be one of the more elegant – and truthful – definitions of psychotherapy.

We hope that readers will feel able to enter into the spirit of our reflection on our various reflections, perhaps seeing something of their own reflections in the interweaving of our own stories. The tale that unfolds may, however, be more about the warp and weft of our respective lives than about any image that is inlaid on these base threads of our experience. Our concern to elucidate something of the essence of the therapeutic relationship may involve us in sacrificing the brighter threads in favour of those that might, more reasonably, provide a suitable ground for the eventual illumination of experience.

Whatever! We leave these finer points of the detail of the tapestry to the main body of the text and to the unpicking of the individual reader. Let the mapping commence.

References

Barker, P. (1999). *The Talking Cures: An Introduction to the Psychotherapies for Health Care Professionals.* NT Books.

Korzybski, A. (1933). *Science and Sanity.* International Non-Aristotleian Library.

McKeown, R. (1941). *The Basic Works of Aristotle.* Random House.

Szasz, T. S. (1987). *Insanity: The Idea and its Consequences.* John Wiley and Sons.

1

The search for healing counsel

The inner voice – the human compulsion when deeply distressed to seek healing counsel within ourselves, and the capacity within ourselves both to create this counsel and to receive it.

Alice Walker

The end of the beginning

Psychotherapy means 'mental healing' – a blend of the Greek root term for the mind (*psyche*) and the Latin for healing (*therapia*). Like many vintage English neologisms, however, psychotherapy has come to mean – as Tweedledum and Tweedledee might have said – exactly what psychotherapists want it to mean. Even those who settle for trying to help people adapt their patterns of behaviour describe themselves as psychotherapists, although healing of the abstraction called the mind may be very far from their own professional minds. The broad church of psychotherapy now unites, at least in the public mind[1], the psychoanalyst and the behaviour therapist, who once were in almost constant dispute over who owned the 'truth' of the human condition, or at least the software for lasting therapeutic change. Such disputes continue, but are largely relegated to the more esoteric corners of academic dialogue. The influence of a market culture and economic rationalism has generated a new neurosis among therapists; how to prove their therapeutic worth in an increasingly competitive health care culture.

Although the parts of the psychotherapeutic story that unfold in this book lie comfortably within that broad church of mind-healing, as will

---

[1]This usage of the term suggests how our 'minds' might be both greater than the sum of our individual parts, and also may be part of something even bigger than ourselves.

become apparent, the story features the combination (and sometimes synthesis) of elements from many of its branches. Indeed, we might describe the psychotherapy that emerged as *ecumenical* were it not for the fact that, as later chapters show, several influences from Eastern thought introduced a transcultural, if not pantheistic, dimension. As we move from the original and necessary focus on what was going on within Bobbie's mind to a broader appreciation of Bobbie's engagement with her world, in a whole sense, the therapy became less and less like the traditional construction of psychotherapy. The sagacious and largely silent therapist, who twiddled a pencil and notepad as the patient emptied her soul along with her tear ducts, was never in evidence. In his place was an often irreverent individual, no less concerned, who was keen to foster the conditions under which Bobbie might find and nurture her own *inner voice*. All too many psychotherapy patients end up adopting the authoritative voice of the therapist. This trick is not too difficult, since many patients have already internalized the voice of some other authority figure – especially a parent. Often, it is the direction or tormenting of this 'voice' that brings the person to therapy.

The American humorist, Garrison Keillor, offers a sad but all too true example (Keiller, 1986):

> Now you call me on the phone to ask 'why don't you ever call us?' … I didn't call because I don't need to talk to you any more. Your voice is in my head, talking constantly from morning till night. I keep the radio on, but I still hear you and will hear until the day I die, when I will hear you say 'I told you so!

The process of socialization involves children, of necessity, accommodating and internalizing (or taking as their own) the influence of belief systems that belong to the world around them. For many patients who come to therapy, the 'problem' is rarely a specific, psychological event, something that has bruised them emotionally, or triggered the development of some life crisis or catalogue of life crises. Often what emerges is a problem with the way the person construes his or her world of experience – how to make sense of all the 'being and doing' that makes up life. The lens through which patients view the world (and their position within it) has been ground by the various influences of significant figures from their past – parents and teachers in particular. Garrison Keillor seems to make light of the way his mother's voice haunts the world inside his head, even challenging the radio to drown her out. He makes, in the process, a powerful point: who owns the voices in our heads? Do they belong to us – are they the voices of 'I'? Or are they mere echoes of the forces that have shaped us – the voices of 'me'? Much of the subtext of therapy involves exploring this simple yet vital question: what is the nature of the relationship between 'I' and 'me'?

Some schools of therapy assume that, having discovered (rather than constructed) some key general principles about 'being and doing', it is the therapist's responsibility to nurture the patient's appreciation of these human truths. In a quite different vein, the American therapist David Reynolds, who has popularized Japanese concepts of therapy in the West, has written of the need to trust reality – to let reality be the teacher (Reynolds, 1985):

> We believe that there is a reality out there calling for our response. It isn't created by our imagination; it doesn't respond directly to what we wish or feel. It responds to what we do. Reality isn't fair or just in any simple, apparent sense. But it does seem to be orderly and more or less under-standable, as we study it. We trust the inner prompting that tells us what needs to be done in the moment. The clarity of this inner voice improves as we listen and respond to it. We learn to distinguish it from the fleeting impulses and thrashing about of undisciplined mental play ... The strength and guidance of our inner prompting gives direction to our lives. Life takes on special meaning as we go about living it attentively.

Although I have practised and taught most of the main schools of psychotherapeutic thought (Barker, 1999), my practice has, over the past decade, more honestly accommodated the values of 'being and doing' that I first began to explore thirty-five years ago. I have grown to appreciate the significance of Reynolds' emphasis on fostering that inner voice through living life attentively. Like Reynolds, Alan Watts had earlier reached a similar conclusion, albeit by approaching the question from a different angle (Watts, 1961). Watts compared Eastern philosophy and religion with Western psychotherapy, concluding that they shared the same goal as Western psychotherapy: effecting a change in consciousness[2]. When I first read Watts thirty-five years ago I har-boured no ambitions to become a psychotherapist, but his analysis seemed not only plausible, but also sensible to the layman within me. However, whereas psychotherapy has traditionally limited its focus to people in manifest distress, Watts pointed out that the oriental philo-sophical traditions – especially Buddhism and Taoism – concerned them-selves with changing the consciousness of normal, socially adjusted people. Moreover, where the Western psychotherapist risks fixating on the 'skin-encapsulated ego' of the individual mind, Eastern thinkers have never distinguished mind from matter, but see everything as one indivisible whole: the reality that David Reynolds repeatedly refers is within us and without us at one and the same time. One of the tricks we have to learn, in living whole lives, is how to accept what seems para-doxical to the traditional, dualistic Western mind. In that sense, modern physics and, latterly, the New Age therapies have taken almost 3000 years

---

[2]Although various influences might be found in the opening out of Western psychotherapy, history will surely conclude that Watts' influence was not only the most original but the most powerful.

to arrive at (or return to) the (w)holistic perspective of the Oriental traditions.

The nature of psychotherapy

We are, however, getting ahead of ourselves. This may be the appropriate point at which to begin this reflection on the process of psychotherapy, by locating ourselves in space and time. Although psychotherapy as a formal practice is little over a hundred years old, with its late modern roots in Freud's psychoanalysis, the kind of 'mental healing', that lies within the craft stretches back to ancient history, through philosopher-priests to the medicine man and magician. It is important to acknowledge the ancient, and indeed cross-cultural, history of psychotherapy, since the effectiveness of psychotherapy – *why* and *how* it works – still has much in common with the ideas of the philosophers of religion and the inter-personal skills of the shaman. Indeed, magical, religious and scientific viewpoints still influence the development of late twentieth century psy-chotherapies, and are simply three different perspectives on the same phenomenon – the *mental distress* brought by the person who becomes the patient[3].

Indeed, although the public is less trusting of the psychotherapist than it once was, we still turn to such authority figures in the expectation that they will 'explain' the inexplicable – especially the mysteries of how we might have become 'who' we are. This is best illustrated, at least in the UK, by the enduring appreciation of programmes such as *In the Psychiatrist's Chair*[4].

Our ambition to understand the workings (metaphorically) of the mind began with Freud over a century ago, and continues today with various attempts to analyse and evaluate the interpersonal processes of helping people understand, resolve or transcend their mental distress, largely through the power of conversation – the *talking cure*.

Although there are many definitions of psychotherapy, we find in its practice the most appropriate definition, since it reveals what can be done in the name of *healing through helping*. The practices include listening, advising, guiding, educating and even influencing the patient.

---

[3]We are conscious that mental health political correctness has largely rejected the traditional term *patient,* especially in favour of the Americanism *client*. However, the Latin root of the term – *cliens* – suggests a subservient and dependent relationship between a *plebian* and a *patron* that seems inappropriate to therapy, which seeks a more egalitarian outcome, if not process.

[4]This is ironic on two counts. The programme illustrates a public misconception that psychiatrists practice psychotherapy, or at least explore the psyches – especially early upbringing and experience. The psychiatrist featured, Professor Anthony Clare, who has so successfully explored the emergent psyches of his famous subjects, has repeatedly made it clear that, in his considered opinion, psy-chotherapy is largely useless save perhaps for cognitive therapy or other brief, problem-solving types of intervention.

Our understanding of psychotherapy has been confused by various ideological disputes over ownership of the title, and a catalogue of 'turf wars' between differing schools. Perhaps, however, the following definition might gain the general approval of psychotherapists:

> Psychotherapy involves the psychological treatment of problems of living, by a trained person, within the context of a professional relationship, involving *either* removing, reducing or modifying specific emotional, cognitive or behavioural problems *and/or* promoting social adaptation, personality development and/or personal growth.

It should not be forgotten, however, that the decision as to whether or not such problems exist, and have or have not been ameliorated, should remain with the patient.

The range of methods that might be employed in such a 'psychological treatment' is virtually limitless, ranging across individual, couple, group and family therapies. All are, however, dependent on some form of interpersonal communication – a conversation between therapist and patient. Many therapies now emphasize their *humanistic* basis, even if not avowedly members of the humanistic school, by aiming to promote some kind of growth in the patient. However, some therapeutic schools, which lie on the periphery of conventional practice, assume that the problem is not one of maturity (or growth) but of wholeness. Such therapies, especially those that are philosophically congruent with Buddhist thought, assume that if the person is striving for anything it is wholeness, and this state is often achieved by encouraging doing less rather than more; by returning the person to his or her 'sacred centre' (Barker, 1999).

The focus of psychotherapy – what people bring to therapy, or what brings them to it – may take various forms: feelings, thoughts or disturbing patterns of behaviour. In general, such problems result in some problem of living[5] that distresses the person, other people, or both. The notion of the 'problem of living' does not deny the influence of biology in the generation of mental distress, but assumes that many more factors other than biology alone are interacting to generate the problem, which is implied by the notion of 'mental illness'. In that sense, a 'problem of living' suggests the whole lived experience of the person, which has long been emphasized by Eastern thought.

The process of psychotherapy requires the fostering and development of a highly specific relationship between patient and therapist, which, unlike ordinary relationships, emphasizes a collaborative undertaking geared toward the attainment of specific therapeutic objectives. To the fly on the wall, it may just sound like two (or more) people talking – a highly

---

[5]This term, which was popularized by Thomas S. Szasz, was first coined by the American psychoanalyst, Harry Stack Sullivan (Sullivan, 1947).

ordinary thing. The sheer ordinariness of the undertaking may belie its extraordinariness.

Some forms of psychotherapy are problem-specific, aiming only to reduce distress or to promote a limited form of social adaptation. Other therapies, especially within the humanistic school, are concerned more with the development of the personality, freeing patients from limiting ways of thinking, feeling or behaving, which restrict the expression of their full humanity. These represent a break from the tradition of therapy as a narrow, medicalized treatment of mental or nervous disorders, and have more in common with the Eastern view that learning 'how to live' is an undertaking for everyone, not simply for those who develop difficulties along the life path. We recognize, however, that for most people in Western societies psychotherapy is more about 'fixing' discrete problems that have emerged in their lives rather than 'learning how to live' in any holistic sense.

Although the usefulness of traditional forms of psychotherapy is difficult to evaluate, at face value most problem-oriented therapies appear to meet their goal of reducing distress. The extent to which the humanistic, and especially the transpersonal therapies, represent a viable alternative to such traditional models remains in doubt. This may have something to do with the all-encompassing, often spiritual, issues that such forms of therapy address. When Freud began to explore the functioning of the mind – as it was understood in late nineteenth century Viennese society – he used the contemporary metaphors of science and technology. Hence the stress given to 'drive mechanisms', 'internal pressure' and 'release valves', illustrative of the science of mechanics that provided the steam engine and would soon produce the engine for the motor car. One hundred years later, those who reflect on the most appropriate metaphors for the workings of the mind are inclined to employ computer terminology. Some even conclude that the neurochemical 'events' that can be traced through the latest scanning device actually represent the formation of thoughts and beliefs, rather than being the 'traces' of our minds at work. *Plus ça change!* Perhaps in another hundred years these metaphors might seem just as naïve as Freud's dynamic representation of the mystery of mental life.

Psychotherapy and psychoanalysis

Although most dictionary definitions include psychoanalysis as one of the psychotherapies, this is misleading. Psychoanalysis involves a systematic and total resolution of unconscious conflicts, and as a result requires structural alteration of defences and character organization (Wolberg, 1995). Clearly this is an ambitious undertaking, requiring a major investment of commitment and time on the part of both therapist and patient. This is the kind of psychotherapy most understood by the general public, especially those reared on classic films like *Suddenly Last Summer*, where Montgomery Clift plays the intense yet caring analyst to Elizabeth Taylor's traumatized and dissociated patient. More recently, the films of Woody Allen have reflected a society where 'being in therapy' was seen as a sign of success, providing that whatever brought the patient to therapy did not stop them earning the good living, necessary to pay for it. Although psychoanalytic ideas and methods are to be found in many forms of psychotherapy, the traditional analysis – with its free association and a couch – is purchased only by a select few. In part this is a function of a gradual loss of faith in the psychoanalytic project, many arguing that psychoanalysis failed to deliver anything approximating a 'talking cure'. However, its demise is more a function of economics, the prohibitive cost of regular, long-term analytic sessions prompting the development of ever briefer (and cheaper) alternatives.

By contrast with psychoanalysis, psychotherapy appears less ambitious, seeking more practical goals resolving discrete problems. Indeed, psychoanalysts might even emphasize the value of encouraging the retention of certain problematic behaviour patterns (such as neurotic defences) if these will allow the person to live life more effectively. This does not mean that psychoanalysis occupies some kind of 'higher ground', or is in any way 'better' than psychotherapy. Given the ambitions of formal psychoanalysis, a stringent selection procedure operates. It is not appropriate for everyone, and indeed certain personality and motivational characteristics are necessary, not to mention the investment of time and (usually) money. Few people might, therefore, be considered appropriate for analysis, whereas just about anyone can be considered for some form of psychotherapy. The critical question is *what* form of therapy?

In establishing psychoanalysis, Freud laid the basis for a highly specific 'school' which required strict observance on the part of its followers. He maintained, to the end of his life, that no one could be an analyst who did not accept the foundation of the theory of psychoanalysis. This meant that an analyst must accept the existence of unconscious mental processes, the theory of repression and resistance and, perhaps most importantly, the importance of sexuality and the Oedipus complex (Freud, 1952). Although various splinter groups within traditional psychoanalysis have developed, it remains a form of human helping quite distinct from the mainstream psychotherapy, and is a world away from the kind of therapy that represented the backdrop to our story. However, Freud's rigid position stimulated – albeit indirectly – the emergence of psychoanalytic or psychodynamic psychotherapy, which accepts some but not all of Freud's original ideas. The position of psychoanalysis, as a preferred method of treatment, belongs to the past. However, this does not mean that its importance as a form of influence or as a means of helping us understand how psychotherapy works has lessened. Indeed, 'psychoanalytically-oriented' or 'psychodynamic' psychotherapy has become arguably the most common form of psychotherapy world-wide. However, many critics, especially those from the 'evidence-based' camp, might wish that this were not the case.

The functions of psychotherapy

The number of practices that might be described as 'psychotherapy' certainly run into hundreds. Twenty years ago, as many as 250 different therapies had been listed (Herink, 1980; Corsini, 1981). Many enjoyed only a short-lived prominence, especially on the West Coast of America. Although there are five key groups of psychotherapy (psychoanalytic, cognitive-behavioural, humanistic, family and solution-focused), for the purpose of this introduction it is worth considering what these might have in common. What are main *functions* of all forms of psychotherapy? Three core functions thread their way through most, if not all, of the psychotherapies: support; re-education; and reconstruction.

Support

Most people who come for therapy[6] experience distress, which they wish to be reduced if not eliminated. These people want to rebalance their emotional equilibrium. They want to develop a sense of control over their circumstances.

Supportive forms of psychotherapy emphasize very specific, often narrow, objectives. The therapist tries to help the person strengthen existing defences, which might offer them the kind of security that will allow them to deal with their difficulties. In providing such support, the therapist has four main options available:

1. *Offering guidance* and *reassurance* – encouraging the person to accept some aspects of his or her experience, while trying to see other parts as a 'necessary evil' at this stage of the person's development
2. *Facilitating emotional catharsis* – allowing (or encouraging) the patient to express feelings, especially strong feelings that have been buried (metaphorically) to date
3. *Promoting self-esteem* – helping the person to identify and clarify personal assets or resources
4. *Enabling coping responses* – helping the person manage specific problems.

Various options are available, from hypnosis, through training in deep

---

[6]Here, this means only those who come voluntarily. People who are 'sent' for therapy represent a quite different scenario.

muscle relaxation, to encouraging group membership, which might provide additional emotional support and, through peer-identification, help to 'normalize' what the person believes is a unique set of problems.

Re-education

Other people want, or need, to make specific changes in the way they live their lives. This may involve fulfilling their creative potential, including their capacity to deal with some problem, or adjusting their goals for everyday living. Such objectives may involve facilitating changes within the person, in their relationships with others, or both.

Re-educative forms of psychotherapy focus directly on changing patterns of living. Although the person may become more insightful or aware of conscious conflicts, this is not always necessary. Depending on the presenting problem of living, any of the following might be offered:

1. *Behaviour* or *conditioning therapy* – changing the specific patterns of a problematic emotion or behaviour, such as reducing anxiety or increasing assertiveness
2. *Client-centred therapy* – developing the patient's self-awareness
3. *Rational–emotive therapy* – focusing on self-defeating beliefs
4. *Marital or family therapy* – addressing specific relationship difficulties
5. *Cognitive therapy* – focusing on unhelpful styles of thinking and acting
6. *Psychodrama* – developing awareness of important life events through re-enactment
7. *Philosophic therapy* (e.g. existential or Zen Buddhist) – setting problems of living within a wider frame of spiritual reference.

Reconstruction

Finally, some people desire, or need, to address their problems of living at a more deep-seated level, aiming to develop insight into unconscious conflicts, making discrete changes to their character structure, or expanding their personality through the development, for them, of some new-found 'human potential'.

Reconstructive therapy implies the need to go 'deeper' into the personality structure. Most, although not all, of the approaches used to accomplish this will be psychoanalytic in form. As noted above, there now exists a great range of 'schools' of analysis – from traditional Freudian psychoanalysis, through various Neo-Freudian approaches, to various psychoanalytical-oriented psychotherapies, including transactional analysis, existential analysis and group analysis.

These approaches may be supplemented by hypnosis or adjunct drug therapy (especially sedation), play therapy in the case of children, and art therapy for those who need to express material that is somehow 'beyond words'.

Counselling and psychotherapy

Although we now use the terms counselling and psychotherapy interchangeably, once these were much more discrete. In *counselling*, patients (usually called 'clients')[7] were helped to understand themselves better so that they might take some action to remedy or resolve some social or adjustment difficulty. This process was usually short-term, and focused on specific difficulties in the 'here and now' of the patient's experience. Traditionally, counsellors offered suggestions about how clients might help themselves, and actively interpreted the patients' feelings and attitudes. This kind of counselling served a supportive function: the counsellor adopted the position of an authority, helping patients to help themselves through evaluating problems and possible courses of action. Psychotherapy had, ostensibly, more complex ambitions, addressing more complex issues involving either re-education or personality reconstruction. The psychotherapist adopted a much less directive function, and the goals were much longer term.

With the development of Rogers' non-directive counselling (Rogers, 1942), the differences between psychotherapy and counselling became blurred. Rogers advocated a careful facilitation of the expression of feelings by the client, within a supportive relationship. The emphasis was, however, on the client undertaking most of the 'work', the counsellor acting as an emotional sounding board and reflecting back the essence of the patient's emotional expression, helping to clarify the form and function of the essentials of the patient's experience. This process aimed at helping clients to assume responsibility for their feelings, and to consider what they needed to do next to address their life problems.

We could take the view that counselling focuses only on resolving specific, situational problems, whereas psychotherapy addresses broader problems – such as personality or esteem difficulties – that *result* in situational crises. This casts counselling as mere 'everyday helpfulness' and psychotherapy as a more heroic style of human intervention. Although such a definition might be workable in vocational or educational counselling, counselling of the bereaved, the dying and others with complex emotional, behavioural and even spiritual problems have all been developed. Although these are everyday problems, they invariably require a heroic gesture of support and intervention. At the same time, some forms of psychotherapy – such as behavioural psychotherapy – can be highly

---

[7]The use of this term was popularized by Carl Rogers in the 1940s in the USA.

specific, aiming to resolve specific emotional or behavioural problems, and no more.

For purely pragmatic reasons, it seems appropriate to use the terms counselling and psychotherapy interchangeably, recognizing that their emphasis will differ according to their supportive, re-educative or reconstructive functions.

The nature of the therapist

All psychotherapy takes place within the context of a highly specific relationship. It may seem ordinary, but it is quite extraordinary. The characteristics of the therapist, and how the process of therapy is managed, play a significant part in its success or failure. Five main therapeutic features are important: good authority; communication; direction; encouragement; and safe space

Good authority

Patients entering therapy are likely to be demoralized, distraught or otherwise 'suffering'. The therapist's primary responsibility is to develop a relationship within which patients may feel emotionally secure, so that they might begin to address the problem that they have brought to therapy. This principle applies whatever the therapeutic aims – supportive, re-educative or reconstructive. Essentially, patients put their destiny in the hands of someone who they hope will be understanding, protective, non-punitive and helpful. Patients hope for these qualities, perhaps because these self-same qualities have been absent in the other significant authority figures in their lives. These essential qualities of 'good authority' preside over the whole therapeutic process.

The greater the distress experienced by the patient, the more likely it is that he or she will represent the therapist as an idealized parent (authority) figure. The nature of this power dynamic – with the therapist very much in charge (control) and the patient dependent on support and approval – can represent a challenge for the therapist, especially with the risk of abusing such power. Some therapists intentionally develop the power dynamic with the patient (especially psychoanalytic therapists), while others try to reduce this, making the relationship more equal and balanced (especially cognitive therapists). However, the differential in power between patient and therapist is central to all psychotherapy. Indeed, by virtue of their expectation that the therapist will be helpful, patients' *project* power (and authority) on to their therapist by assuming, quite appropriately, that he or she will be an 'authority on the patient's problems' and will be able to help to ameliorate them. However, the fundamental and powerful nature of this union allows the therapist to restore the patient's morale. The restoration of morale is one of the core functions of all the psychotherapies (Frank, 1974).

Communication

Therapy is no more than a conversation developed within an extraordinary relationship. The therapist tries to help patients grow by developing their understanding of the nature of their problem. To do so, the therapist needs to be able to communicate in terms that are not only understandable to patients – couched in their own language – but also acceptable, given the stage of emotional development they have reached.

In addition to knowing *what* to tell the patient, and *how* to frame this, the therapist also needs to know *when* it would be appropriate to communicate this. Needless to say, the therapist also needs to know when it would be politic to keep his counsel.

Direction

The therapist may be involved in helping patients to establish the meaning of certain experiences, chart their own course, or determine what actions need to be taken. Throughout these various manoeuvres, direction is always being provided. Ironically, even by being 'non-directive', the therapist provides direction of some sort. Such direction is expected. If patients were able to work out things for themselves, they would not have come to therapy.

Encouragement

The therapist also serves as a source of encouragement, helping patients become aware of progress, reinforcing their independent decision-making, and helping them to stay focused on dealing with problems and issues that they might otherwise wish to turn away from. This appears simple. However, offering support and encouragement to people with many years of experience of self-criticism or even self-hatred can be a tall order.

Safe space

In most forms of psychotherapy, patients need to reflect on attitudes, values or beliefs – about themselves or others – that they have long held, considering their origins and considering other ways of construing the world. This involves people looking (metaphorically) at themselves in a 'full-length mirror', perhaps even 'naked'. If it involves nothing else, therapy involves a metaphorical form of undressing, often stripping down to the very core of the person's emotional being. People can only undertake such challenging personal work successfully when they have reached a certain stage in the relationship. Time limits cannot be put on this. It may take a few sessions, or many more. However, this 'safe space' grows out of the good authority with which the relationship began, and also represents a crucial stage in the closure of the relationship.

Trusting to fate – expecting a change for the better

The five 'therapeutic gifts' described above are found in all effective therapy. They represent the processes that operate in all 'human helping', whether or not we call it psychotherapy. Carl Rogers attached a new set of terms to some of these dimensions of the therapeutic relationship, emphasizing the need for *warmth*, *empathy*, *genuineness* and *unconditional positive regard*. These apparently simple characteristics of the therapist's orientation towards the patient provide the basis for the restoration of basic trust, which is the central task of psychotherapy (Strupp, 1972).

Not all therapists emphasize the importance of the relationship to the same extent. Some suggest that the relationship merely supports the application of specific psychotherapy techniques. Such a view is often favoured by behavioural or cognitive psychotherapists (Newell and Dryden, 1991). For other therapists, the relationship is central. What produces the results is the dedication of the therapist to a specific system, the sincerity of purpose – the transmission of a message to the patients that the therapist 'cares' about what happens to them (Rogers, 1965).

These relationship factors influence the operation of *faith* – the extent to which therapists believe in their chosen method, and the extent to which they can encourage patients to join them. Faith in the therapeutic system can result in therapy working, literally, 'like a charm'. All forms of therapy – physical and psychological – possess placebo properties. The patient's belief in the method, or the therapist's strong 'selling' of the method, produce effects that may have nothing to do with the method itself. Here, modern therapy hearkens back to the power of the shaman: the magic of the psychotherapist still is an important part of the therapeutic process.

Today, there is great emphasis on trying to establish what specific processes in psychotherapy account for specific outcomes. What does the therapist *do*, which produces specific change in the patient's presentation? It appears, at present, that rather than any one thing (or even collection of things), it is more *how* the therapist orchestrates the therapeutic process that determines a good result.

An overview of the therapeutic process

The therapeutic process has four main stages – a beginning, two central stages and a conclusion. Although any analysis of effective therapy will invariably show these stages, they are rarely discrete, and usually overlap. In the *beginning* stage the therapist focuses on establishing a working alliance with the patient. This involves:

- Encouraging the patient to join therapy
- Offering some explanation of what will happen in the process
- Showing understanding of the patient's plight and promoting an appreciation that the therapist will be of some help in addressing this
- Encouraging a preliminary statement of the aims (goals) of the therapy.

In the first of the *central* stages, the therapist explores the background to the patient's problems and the present consequences in everyday life. This involves:

- Exploring the patient's relationship with the problem – seeking to clarify particular thoughts, feelings and actions which are, in some way, *connected* to the problem.

How that 'connection' is explored is determined by the therapist's chosen method. For example, psychoanalytic therapists will probe for unconscious conflicts through use of, for example, free association or dream interpretation; cognitive therapists will look for signs of self-defeating thoughts that might precipitate negative feelings; and behaviour therapists will attempt to identify the specific factors that appear to reinforce dysfunctional patterns of behaviour.

In the second *central* stage, the therapist begins the process of translating the patient's understanding of the problem into action for change, correction of forward movement. Again, a range of options is possible, depending on the method of therapy used. The therapist might:

- Review incentives for change
- Help the patient to manage specific emotional disturbance
- Focus on forces that appear to block the process of change
- Encourage the expression of powerful emotions (catharsis)
- Help the patient to become reconciled to situations which are beyond control.

In the final or *termination* stage, the therapist draws both the process of therapy and the relationship to some kind of a conclusion. Although the patient may have made great strides during the previous three stages, here he or she has to address the complex issue of 'life beyond therapy'.

Irrespective of their ideological persuasion, all therapists have to address similar problems:

- How to bring a necessarily 'dependent' relationship to an end with minimum emotional trauma?
- How to assist the patient to take full ownership of the problem, and the continuing work necessary to maintain, or develop progress in addressing it?
- How to promote the patient's independence and emotional assertiveness beyond therapy, encouraging the patient to recognize how he or she *owns* the full range of experience – problems and successes, highs and lows?

These three stages present all therapists, but especially the novice, with great challenges. In the beginning stage, therapists often find it difficult to relate appropriately to the patient, becoming either irritated by the patient's apparent inability to respond, or lacking any sense of sympathy (far less empathy) for the patient's predicament. Alternatively, therapists may show too much concern, swamping patients with compassion and making them unnecessarily dependent. Roger's ideal of 'non-possessive warmth' can be difficult to judge.

In the central stages, the therapist may avoid addressing patients' problems that, perhaps unconsciously, stimulate anxiety in the therapist.

Alternatively, the therapist may probe too deeply into issues that concern the therapist, but which are not really important to the patient. Again, the patient's 'slowness' or 'resistance' may irritate the therapist; alternatively, the therapist may do too much work, further increasing the dependency of the patient.

In the termination stage, the therapist may find it difficult to 'let go' of the patient. At the conclusion, the parting may be difficult for both therapist and patient, and the therapist may tend to underestimate the patient's capacity for independence or alternatively try to push an ill-prepared patient into a potentially dangerous state of independence.

Therapeutic assignments

Although most therapists encourage patients to 'work' on their problems between sessions – at least encouraging them to think about them – the idea of the formal 'homework assignment', is fairly recent (Ellis, 1962). Assignments became popular within cognitive and behavioural psychotherapies, but are now found in almost all approaches, especially those employing some kind of self-management. The range of assignments is virtually limitless, but they usually emphasize the independent management of the problems that brought the patient to therapy. In most cases patients are encouraged to keep daily logs or diaries recording their thoughts, feelings and actions, and this format may provide the basis for projecting into the future, developing the resolution of the problem.

Patients are usually given an assignment that is related directly to the current work of the session. This may be highly specific or more diffuse. Among the many classic 'diffuse' assignments are the following *practice* assignments:

- Let go of the past
- Tolerate a certain amount of anxiety
- Tolerate a certain degree of hostility
- Tolerate a certain degree of irritation, frustration or deprivation
- Make a small change 'for the better' to your environment
- Identify something that cannot be changed and 'accept it'
- Use your 'will power' to stop engaging in some destructive activity
- Challenge one negative view of yourself
- Select a pleasurable activity from a list and engage in it
- Make more 'reasonable' demands on yourself
- Accept the responsibilities of your social role, one by one.

The 'golden hour' of therapy can be all too easily overvalued. What does the patient do in the other 167 hours of the week? The homework assignment tries, strategically, to locate the emphasis of therapy in the life of the patient. The consultation serves an important purpose, but perhaps is no more important than a coach sitting down with a player on the edge of the sportsfield to review her performance, and to discuss optional moves or manoeuvres. The athlete did not suddenly arrive at this particular consultation with the coach, but has been working toward this through years of ambition and application. The coach knows that he cannot *produce* a great athlete, but can only use his knowledge of sports and athletes in general to draw out from within (*educe*) some of the key experiences of *this particular athlete*, which she might use to reshape her ambition and revise her application.

This coaching analogy seems wholly appropriate to the field of psychotherapy. The coach needs to get very close to the athlete, gaining her confidence so that he might step (metaphorically) into her world of experience, so that he can review, along with her, the various dimensions of her performance. However, the coach does not 'take over' the experience of the athlete. The coach may be passionate and will often provoke and challenge the athlete, but this is an 'enacted passion', aiming to facilitate awareness in the athlete – awareness of some 'eternal truth' that the coach already knows only too well.

What future for co-operative therapy?

Although the therapeutic relationship described in this book began modestly, following fairly conventional psychotherapeutic lines, it soon switched tracks to signal the coach–athlete relationship[8]. Such an approach would not be appropriate for all patients. Therapy may share something in common with cooking. When preparing a meal for someone we take note of the general rules of 'good nutrition', not forgetting the specifics of individual dietary requirements, the influences of any 'special occasion', cultural influences and, not least, the vagaries of personal preference. A successful meal is, invariably, a function of the cook, chef or host(ess) recognizing and addressing these different 'needs'. The idea of a universally 'good' menu would be laughable, and certainly unappetizing. However, when it comes to meeting the often disparate human needs that represent themselves in patienthood, especially when collapsed together under some general diagnostic category, therapists continue to pursue the holy grail of a general 'menu' of psychotherapeutic treatment. This may simply lose the individual 'diner' in the process. If we seek to meet the unique needs of the unique individual who is the patient, then we need to develop the therapeutic menu in accordance with the expressed (or implied) needs, wants and wishes of that individual.

If the therapy that is described in the following chapters illustrates any one thing, it is the spirit of therapeutic collegiality: the active pursuit of the processes that might meet the needs of the individual patient. Enough has been written in the closing years of the twentieth century about collaboration and co-operation in therapy and research (Heron, 1996) to suggest that the further development of the 'working alliance', will be the primary focus of therapy in the twenty-first century. We hope that the account of therapy that follows will contribute in some small way to the clarification of the need for an 'individual psychotherapy', which acknowledges at the same time that we are all more simply human than otherwise.

References

Barker, P. (1999). *Talking Cures: A Guide to the Psychotherapies for Health Care Professionals.* NT Books.

Corsini, R. J. (1981). *Handbook of Innovative Psychotherapies.* John Wiley and Sons.

Ellis, A. (1962). *Reason and Emotion in Psychotherapy.* Lyle Stuart.

Frank, J. D. (1974). Psychotherapy: the restoration of morale. *Am. J. Psychiatry*, **16**, 271–4.

Freud, S. (1952). Postscript to a discussion on lay analysis. In: *Collected Papers*, Vol. 5, pp. 205–14. Hogarth Press.

Herink, R. (1980). *The Psychotherapy Handbook.* The New American Library.

---

[8]Although I have popularized this conception of therapy, it is an old idea, articulated first – to my knowledge – by Michael Mahoney (Mahoney, 1974).

Heron, J. (1996). *Co-operative Inquiry: Research into the Human Condition.* Sage.

Keiller, G. (1986). *Lake Woebegone Days.* Faber and Faber.

Mahoney, M. J. (1974). *Cognition and Behaviour Modification.* Ballinger.

Newell, R. and Dryden, W. (1991). Clinical problems: an introduction to the cognitive behavioural approach. In: *Adult Clinical Problems: A Cognitive Behavioural Approach* (W. Dryden and R. Rentoul, eds), p. 4. Routledge.

Reynolds, D. (1985). *Playing Ball on Running Water.* Sheldon Press.

Rogers, C. (1942). *Counselling and Psychotherapy: Newer Concepts in Practice.* Houghton and Mifflin.

Rogers, C. (1965). *Client-centred Therapy.* Houghton and Mifflin.

Strupp, H. H. (1972). On the technology of psychotherapy. *Arch. Gen. Psychiatry,* **26,** 270–78.

Sullivan, H. S. (1947). *Conceptions of Modern Psychiatry.* William Alanson White Foundation.

Watts, A. W. (1961). *Psychotherapy East and West.* Pantheon Books.

Wolberg, L. (1995). *The Technique of Psychotherapy,* 4th edn. Jason Aronson Inc.

2

Life as drama

For a long time it seemed to me that life was about to begin – real life. But there was always some obstacle in the way, something to be got through first, some unfinished business, time still to be served, a debt to be paid. Then life would begin. At last it dawned on me that these obstacles were my life.

Fr Alfred D'Souza

Introduction

The players, the stage and the unfolding script

What we shall speak of as 'therapy' here involves a tour of the patient's life. In the process, we are required to traverse some of the terrain of the therapist. We hope to show how the metaphor of the *grand tour* that therapy often can become may, of itself, become a *journey*. It should also become clear how that journeying, moment by moment, day by day and, not infrequently, night by sleepless night, can become synonymous with discovery.

We shall explore how the patient journeyed to the therapist's door; what struggles had already been witnessed; and what kind of shape – metaphorically speaking – she was in at the start and how that shape changed.

Shakespeare's children

It may seem trite to remind ourselves of the human drama that lies at the heart of every story related in therapy. However, we often take the status of the 'play' too lightly, failing to appreciate the layers of complexity that lie within, and perhaps beyond, the script. As we struggle for success and recognition in our lives, we forget that life is a game to be played. Indeed, as Plato observed, life *must* be lived as play, using 'play' in its broadest sense. In considering the status of Shakespeare's plays, Driscoll wondered about what was going on (Driscoll, 1983):

> And what is the ontological status of a character or a play? An imitation of life? A partaker of life? Or a vision of life?

Although for many of us the soap opera now dominates the cultural map of the human interior, even those plays on our emotions are the embodiment of the vagaries of all our lives. There we find echoes of our own experience, misery and despair, but less so our joys and liberation. The designation of the play as drama was clearly no accident. Shakespeare would have been very much at home with the gritty realism of *Brookside* or *Eastenders*, plays that, like his own, emphasize moral and ethical dilemmas – often at the expense of fact or continuity.

The same lack of fact and continuity often threads through our own narratives. The words of the drama play, through a musical metaphor, on our heart strings, plucking and bending the sounds of our deepest experiences, even when they reflect nothing more than the foibles of everyday living. The strange power the stories *of* our lives have *over* our lives carries a brutal fascination, especially perhaps when they reflect our human ordinariness. Words will, for this reason, be writ large in the account that unfolds here. The extent to which we write our own script or co-create it, albeit unconsciously, through our dialogue with others, remains unclear to many of us, and may even be beyond the understanding of the person who becomes a patient. For as soon as she has begun to think of herself as a patient, she will likely have begun to think that some mysterious dramatist has scripted not only all of her words, but the moves in her relations with self and others. The surrender of *personhood* to the domination of *patienthood* rarely leaves much room for negotiation.

If there is one thing that the play captures, which satisfies most of us (at least when it works) and proves the enduring attraction of theatre, it is the suggestion of the spiritual realm within us all. In an interview with the Shakespearean actor Mark Rylance, the psychiatrist Rob Ferris noted (Ferris, 1992):

> There is a workaday sense in which we look at people's experiences and try to categorize them fairly crudely and bluntly as normal or abnormal, as part of the process of diagnosing mental illness and deciding about treatment. Perhaps it might be said that this process actively avoids the spiritual aspects or dimension which something like the play taps.

This observation touched a nerve in the actor, prompting him to consider how he had come to understand the nature of the 'irrational' in some of Shakespeare's characters:

> Perhaps that's why there are so many books written about Hamlet; yet none of them could explain what some of the lines meant. It took me 80 or 90 performances before I learned what some of them meant. There is no way you can do it with a dictionary or rational thought. It is only through play that you get there.

Again, it seems trite to observe that, despite the burgeoning literature on the whole complex continuum of human experience from outright madness through to more everyday doubts about our sanity, all these stories are, in a sense, epiphenomenal; they float, often vicariously, around and about the human experience. Perhaps our greatest mistake has been to believe that some wise person actually could know us better than we know ourselves. The trick performed, often artlessly, by therapists of different persuasions has been to feign knowledge. The knowledge expressed by therapists is no more than a play upon the story expressed by the patient, who without necessarily knowing it has been unpacking the wisdom of her soul, chapter by chapter, sometimes line by painful line. The epistemological challenge – how can I *know* that I know – faced by the patient is often so great that it seems easier to surrender to the packaged epistemology of the therapist. He will tell her what she needs to know *and* how she might come to know it. Whether this collusion is recognized on either side is of little consequence. That seems to be the substance of our faith in therapy and therapists. Why else should we revere someone who does little more than recycle our words and tune-up their inherent wisdom?

Writing and re-authoring

Therapy is pretty much like any other form of storytelling – it has a beginning, a middle, and something that serves (at least for the time being) as an end. As soon as we speak from the heart, we all become Shakespeare's children. Your story begins way past the end, in the sense that you are now more than seven years further down the road from where we parted. Your story is told largely from that perspective – looking back down the road you have travelled. I say *largely*, for the script that unfolds here does not just involve the detailed and highly evocative records of your many experiences of therapeutic travel, which are now history, but also your consideration of what these mean for us both now. As you refer to these contemporary accounts, you reconstruct (and at the same time deconstruct) the psychotherapy traveller's tale. What you were largely unaware of as you wrote those long epistles, week after week, was that you were carefully re-authoring your own life. Not *editing* it, embellishing the positive bits and excising the pain and suffering. Rather, you were engaging with the powerful metaphors embedded in those journal notes and letters. Each engagement generated a new line of thought, pursued by reflection, resulting in another record. Your personal notes, accounts of your homework assignments and letters followed on naturally from the telling of the tale within the session. They became a kind of reprise of the essentials of that experience.

When I asked one of my mentors, Hildegard E. Peplau (1901–1999) how, in her view, people came to 'be', she said 'people make themselves up as they talk'. The wisdom of those simple words are the first and last post of the fence of therapy, over which therapists hang eagerly in their efforts to relate to the patient on the other side. And of course people talk to themselves covertly, as they think aloud and, most powerfully, when they commit those thoughts to paper in exactly the way you illustrated. We have no need of Shakespeare as an amanuensis when we can draft and redraft the saga of our lives, each word illuminating the last one, even when it appears to suggest a confused path leading to a dead end.

The impatient patient: symptoms and dis-ease

I had very clear goals when I entered therapy. I wanted to stop rising six feet in the air when the phone on my desk rang. I wanted to be able to read and remember what I had read without returning repeatedly to the same text and repeatedly failing to retain the contents. I wanted eight hours uninterrupted sleep each night. I wanted to stop breaking out in a cold sweat for no apparent reason, watching my hands shake uncontrollably. I wanted to be able to enjoy a night at home with my own company, or a visit to friends, instead of running out of my house because I couldn't bear to be alone; then leaving five minutes after I arrived at a friend's house because I couldn't bear to be in company either. I wanted to lose the crushing weight that pressed on my chest and the rapidly beating heart that frequently made me feel light-headed and blanche. Most disabling of all were the battles for breath that could last for several hours, with me eventually locked in some kind of coma-like state where I was barely aware of what was going on around me.

In those days the world was a threatening place. I looked at everyone who was dear to me and wondered if it was the last time I would ever see them, worried that a car accident might crush their life away or medical science be overwhelmed by a sudden invader who leaves loved ones cold and dead. Psychotic rapists lurked round every corner, haunting my waking hours and my sleeping. Every time I put the key in the lock of my door, I had visions of finding the disorder of a burglar's visit.

I didn't want a therapist who would ignore the very disabling symptoms, fixing on the search for the root causes of my anxiety. I wanted somebody to make the symptoms go away and let me get on with my life. Ultimately that somebody was me, but if I'd really believed that at the start I would have been terrorized and suffered an increase in the severity of the symptoms.

Arrivals: finding an appropriate therapist

I am conscious that I use the word helpful now when describing successful therapeutic techniques and learned personal skills. In the beginnings of therapy, I was obsessed with what was 'right' and what was 'wrong'. But what was 'right' for me at one stage wouldn't necessarily be 'right' for me three months down the line. The sort of free-ranging exploration that went on during the latter stages of therapy would have been unworkable in the early stages, when I paced the room and couldn't face the therapist, let alone speak about the terrors that so consumed me. All I know for sure is that at particular stages, particular approaches and particular suggestions were helpful.

The main purpose of collaborating on this book is to give therapists some idea of what was helpful to me as a person in a therapeutic relationship, and what was unhelpful. Hopefully, these accounts of my experience will also be helpful to people who are either in therapy or might some day need therapy. I am concerned that I might appear overly critical, or even bitter, regarding therapy that was unhelpful. I am mindful of the fact that what might have been unhelpful to me could work a treat for someone else. If some or much of what I have to say appears negative, I make the excuse that much of what was helpful in my therapeutic encounters was absorbed unconsciously, though there were many lightning flashes of insight along the way. When a particular approach or suggestion was very unhelpful, it is more memorable and tends to be highlighted as I look back.

But there has to be a starting point for this private investigation. My first meeting with you would seem like a good point, except that so many of our early therapeutic encounters were shaped by two other therapeutic relationships. Much of what I know to have been helpful in your approach has been understood through contrast and comparison with unsuccessful therapeutic encounters.

I don't think it's necessary to bare my soul and get bogged down in the minutiae of the life problems that gave birth to my disabling anxiety. However, some history is necessary to help the reader appreciate the huge hurdles you had to cross before I gained the confidence to make a leap of faith in you and begin the really exciting work of exploring the limitless self.

Presenting myself for therapy with you was one of the biggest risks I have ever taken. The situation had more than one precedent, and had previously resulted in disaster. Once again I felt like I was teetering on the edge of an abyss, and the choice was to fall over or jump in.

For a number of years I had been experiencing the symptoms of anxiety, though I was only aware of the symptoms and not that they were the manifestation of anxiety. The symptoms troubled me to different degrees at different times, and when I was severely affected I had no words to describe what I believed to be a freakish experience unique to myself. I used the expression 'throwing a wobbler', which seemed to cover these terrifying occurrences.

Friends had tried to help, but always found themselves completely out of their depth when they got close enough to see the true extent of my problems. Professional help was advised, but I was never ready to make such a step, which I feared would threaten my job and brand me as a 'mental' case for the rest of my life.

Then I was urged to see a private counsellor – someone I could visit in my own time and who did not fill out formal documents that would follow me through life as part of a permanent health record, alerting every subsequent health practitioner to the possibility that any aches or pains complained of might be 'all in the mind'. This was the great attraction, and I committed myself to what became an expensive period of counselling which lasted almost two years and, tragically, left me more troubled than when I began.

Life events did undoubtedly play a part in my anxious state, but when I presented for treatment in the NHS psychiatric system my problems had already been exacerbated following the sudden collapse of my previous therapeutic relationship with a relatively untrained private counsellor. At the time I experienced his sudden withdrawal as worse than death. Not only was I abandoned forever, but I was abandoned through choice. This man had bitten off more than he could chew, and when he finally admitted he couldn't help I was left more deeply untrusting than before and with absolutely no faith in my ability to judge other people or their capacity to help or hurt me. This was a man who, over a 21-month period of therapy, I had come to depend upon, who I thought I knew and knew me. Yet having dragged me screaming to the darkest corners of my being, he fled, leaving me teetering on the edge of an abyss.

The disabling symptoms of breathless panting, sweating, trembling and sleeplessness that had led me to the private counsellor became worse, and I finally went to the GP. This was her first indication there was a mental health problem. Within six weeks I had a referral to the psychiatric outpatient clinic. There began several months of therapeutic intervention with a consultant psychiatrist who practised as a psychoanalyst. It was to be a frustrating experience for both of us.

With hindsight, I must have been deeply insulting to this traditionally qualified lady, frequently making comparisons with the private counsellor. He was a man who had a day job and fitted in his private counselling work on evenings and at weekends. Basically he had undergone marriage

guidance training, but after studying a short course based on the tech-
niques of Carl Rogers he set up as a 'person-centred therapist". Hardly
a match for a physician who had become a psychiatrist and then spe-
cialized as an analyst.

One of the biggest stumbling blocks to establishing a relationship with
the psychiatrist was that the private counsellor had picked up a certain
amount of psychobabble and technique, which I reacted against when I
found an echo in the professional psychiatrist. The concerned gaze, the
'reassuring' pat on the arm and the repeated 'mmms' were a constant
reminder of that earlier failed relationship. Far from serving as a prod to
unravel the troubled workings of my mind, they frequently made me dry
up in terror as I saw myself ending at the same impasse as in the earlier
therapeutic relationship.

More terrifying for me was the lack of eye contact. Often when I looked
at the psychiatrist to gauge how what I had said was being received, all
I saw was a bowed head as she made copious notes. I had the unwar-
ranted but very real feeling that everything I said was being taken down
and would be used in evidence to label me a straitjacket case. I did not
respond well to the psychoanalytic therapy on offer. I experienced my
sessions with the psychiatrist as oppressive silences which I felt com-
pelled to fill with I knew not what. Several times she told me it was my
hour to talk about whatever I wanted, but I couldn't respond. I couldn't
find a way into a meaningful soliloquy. Often I felt like shouting, 'If I
knew what to do myself, I wouldn't be asking you for help'. I was looking
for some magic trick that would make it all okay.

The long silences I felt compelled to fill had been a feature of my rela-
tionship with the private counsellor. The whole sorry mess of that thera-
peutic relationship no longer has the power to hurt me, but maybe it
needs to be set down to help the reader understand why I arrived at
certain views on therapy.

I clearly remember the 'last straw' that broke the camel's back and
drove me to seek the private counsellor's help. I had been having some
pretty bad wobblers for some time, but they had been getting more fre-
quent and more intrusive and I, as a consequence, had been making more
demands on friendships than friendship can easily bear. For some time a
particular friend had been urging me to consult the counsellor, and after
a particularly distressing experience at work I called him and asked for
an appointment. He made one for that very afternoon.

Looking back, I realize how important the surroundings of the con-
sulting room are for putting the client at ease and creating the environ-
ment wherein they feel comfortable telling their story. The first thing I set
eyes on when I walked into the room was a box of tissues, sitting in splen-
did isolation on a low, round table in the centre of the room. I was freaked
at the thought that I was expected to snivel in front of this complete
stranger. I can't tell you how intrusive and upsetting I found that box of
tissues. However, at future meetings I asked to have it removed, and even-

tually it was nearly always cleared away before I arrived or the counsel-
lor grabbed it and put it out of sight as he showed me in for an appoint-
ment. At that first meeting I paced up and down, unable to sit in one spot
and face him. I also had a severely dry mouth and felt unable to speak,
literally as if I had dried up. I didn't throw a wobbler at that first meeting,
but I was able to give him some idea of what happened. Later he was to
write that he had never encountered such a 'phenomenon' before in all
his years of counselling.

One friend takes the view, perhaps uncharitably, that his clients were
all bored housewives with plenty of cash whose husbands didn't have
time to talk to them. Real mental health problems, he hadn't encountered.
With hindsight I think that is possibly partly true, but he did tell me he
had counselled people who had suffered similar life events. In all his
years of counselling, I was the only person he was forced to drop.

I found appointments very difficult because I didn't know what to say,
and also experienced as a physical, threatening presence all the bad
things that might come out if I could start to speak. It would take me
three-quarters of an hour to settle and start to talk, and I'd no sooner
started than time was up.

About the third or fourth appointment, I had a really bad wobbler. The
appointment was in the early evening, and it was close on midnight when
I left. I don't remember anything except coming to, with my friend sitting
on the counsellor's study floor cradling my head in her lap. I had thrown
a wobbler and he didn't know what to do, so he had phoned my friend. I
was so distressed, I wasn't thinking or feeling anything that night. I sent
him £70 for the appointment (it cost £15 an hour to see him). When I
think about it now it was a rip-off, because although undoubtedly I had
disrupted his whole evening, it was my friend who had all the work, and
shouldered all the responsibility. She should have got the fee!

I really was a genuine pain in the neck, and made the guy's life hell.
As soon as we got anywhere approaching a difficult topic, I would start
running scared and bail out into a wobbler. This was a really serious
problem for him. First, he didn't know what to do with me – whether it
was best to leave me 'til I came out of it or to stay with me (though since
I was largely unaware of anything that was going on around me in that
state, that seemed a waste of his time). I was also a logistical nightmare.
Many times he complained, quite legitimately, that he was unable to book
other appointments on evenings when he saw me because I would spill
long over the hour.

Very early in our therapeutic relationship I asked if I could have two-
hour appointments(£30 a week crippled me until I was literally selling
heirlooms). That way I was able to settle down at the start and get going.
But this became a problem. It was a 'boundary' I had imposed, and one
of the ways he felt I was taking 'control'. He was concerned by my need
to remain in control. However, I still believe this was a reasonable desire
on my part, given that I was expected to continue functioning in society

during the period of therapy and my disabling symptoms, which were worrying myself and others, represented a complete lack of control and left me very vulnerable. In that state I could not take care of myself – an absolute loss of control.

Then I discovered that the counsellor thought I was trying to control him. This is very interesting, because the evidence he quoted were measures I took to CONTROL MYSELF in a bid to get the optimum benefit from therapy. He always offered coffee at the start of a session, real coffee. I didn't think this was good for me, because one of the symptoms I was trying to eradicate was an overactive startle response. Anyone who can read a tabloid knows that caffeine makes you jumpy. However I did, as I've said, have a problem with drying up, so I asked to have a glass of water. I always carried a straw during this period as I had cut my mouth when my jaw went into spasm as I was trying to have a drink during a wobbler. At this time I would often have wobblers alone in bed, and I discovered I could get fluid in at times when I was slipping into or out of the wobbler if I used a straw. It seemed a very simple solution to the problem.

Because I knew I was having difficulty settling during therapy and controlling my anxiousness, I tried to find ways to reduce the symptoms of my anxiety. I thought at the time, and still do, that I was trying to find positive steps to help myself and to help the counsellor help me. He complained that he couldn't do his work if I didn't talk to him. That was fair enough. Surely it was fair enough for me to try and find a way to let him work?

I discovered a relaxation technique in a book, for which the person trying to relax needed the help of a reader to recite a list of images for visualization. I asked the counsellor if we could start our session with that. He obliged, and I was amazed at how much better our session went as a result. I really was very relaxed. The next week I asked to start the same way, and for several weeks we started each session with fifteen minutes relaxation.

About six months into counselling, the counsellor asked me if I would like to read his notes. After each session he would record what had happened, and his thoughts. I was intrigued and apprehensive at the same time, but took the notes. It was there that I read how he was irritated by all the things I did to control him; these were his words. He cited the relaxation exercises, the glass of water and my often deciding to sit on the floor in a corner (where I felt more comfortable). I still maintain that these were things I did to control my own disruptive behaviours, not to control him. Anyway, that was it. I stopped doing these things, because by then I was hooked and wanted to please him.

The other thing I really reacted to in the counsellor's notes was his mentioning a colleague who had been trying to get him to drop me because I was 'a bottomless case'. This is important, because it had an effect on a subsequent exchange with my psychiatrist. I stormed back to the counsellor and asked who this guy was. He had stressed at the start how his work was confidential and he wouldn't share my secrets with anyone. Then suddenly this other counsellor appeared. He explained that all counsellors have a supervisor – 'He is your protection as well as mine'. I must admit these words have a pretty hollow ring now. This other counsellor became a real problem for me during therapy. I felt I was fighting an unknown foe, who really didn't like me and wanted my counsellor to dump me. Twelve months before he eventually did dump me, the counsellor assured me that he was his own man and that he didn't always agree with everything his supervisor said. Neither did he always follow his advice. Maybe my life would have been a lot easier in the long run if he had.

Later, the analyst took exception to a comment I made about her telling her supervisor about my bizarre behaviour. She had a rare moment of liveliness, and snapped 'I'm a consultant psychiatrist. I don't have a supervisor'. I can see now that my comment was highly insulting to her, particularly as she was being compared to a bogus professional. But at the time I had no intention of being insulting, and had a genuine concern to find out how far I could trust her, what the system was, etc. But we had a real communication problem. I believe that as individuals we interpret all new experiences according to our experiences of the past. If those experiences have been wildly different from those of the general population, our interpretations will be different, isolating us from our peers. I really wanted to make therapy with the analyst work, because I wanted to be like everybody else and be less freakish. I thought she was my only chance to do that. I realize now that it was always going to be difficult, given all that had gone before. I just think there were times we could have made more sense of each other if she'd been more angled at where I was coming from, rather than following a rigid technical approach with an apparently rigid interpretation of certain behaviours and thoughts of mine.

A good example is the 'mmm' repetition, which was particularly distressing for me because it was a technique of the counsellor. I explained that I found it distressing and why. Surely it wouldn't have been too difficult to say a few words (even non-committal, reassuring noise-type words), given that I had taken the first risk and exposed why I didn't like this technique. She continued to say 'mmm'.

I hope I'm not giving the impression that the counsellor was an ogre, because he wasn't. In time I became deeply attached to him. He was one of the first truly gentle men I have known. At least that is how I came to see him. But even I was concerned that I was becoming too attached to him. The whole point of therapy for me was to learn how to cope alone; instead I was having nightmares about him being killed in a car crash and me being left less able to cope than I was before. I felt I needed him, and that made me feel vulnerable. We even discussed this, and the counsellor assured me it was quite normal for a client to feel dependent on a therapist. He expected this; furthermore he said, 'This is the burden I accept when I take on a case'. I believed him and stopped worrying about it.

The real difficulty for me was that the problem I took to him in the first instance, the wobblers, wasn't getting any better through seeing the counsellor. Eighteen months on they were getting, if anything, worse, as, trusting him totally, I was beginning to open up some of the real sewers of my life. After one particularly bad experience during a session at his house, I just about drove my car off the road because I was in no fit state to be at the wheel. Also I was disturbed that his wife and children could hear me. He said it didn't upset them, but it upset and embarrassed me. After that he started coming to my house so he could just leave if I threw a wobbler.

His coming to my house, in a sense, took me right back to square one. As I said, environment is important, and there is a sense when you go somewhere for therapy that you leave a lot of stuff in the place where it erupted. I was very resistant to opening the sewers in my own front room, my relax-and-watch-TV-here-you-are-safe place. Anyway, it obviously wasn't working for him, and one day he came for a session and announced that he had decided it would be the last. I shouted, cried, threw things. He sat still, said nothing, and after an hour took his £15 and left. I now wonder, where was the 'equality' in that? He was always telling me he didn't lead, he was a volunteer to walk BESIDE me through the dark valleys. But I wasn't consulted at all on the ending, and I had absolutely no safety net. He said he was concerned I was a 'psychotic'. That was an expensive diagnosis. If he really thought that, I would've been in real danger – but he just walked out. It seems, with hindsight, to be very dangerous having one person working alone with no system of being able to refer on if he's not helping. This was the strength of the NHS system. The analyst was clearly making little headway with me, but had an awareness of the work of a number of mental health practitioners and an ability to refer on to an appropriate therapist. Though the analyst has reason to wish I had never darkened her doorstep, I will forever be grateful to her for identifying someone who was interested in simply 'helping' me.

Soul-work and power

You have introduced us to some of the important players in the therapeutic drama – the counsellor, the analyst, the therapist (myself) and, not least, yourself. There was also a fourth player, a psychologist, who will appear in a later chapter, but for now these four represent the core of the cast.

Your summary of the process that led you to my door has been stripped of much of the emotional flesh, which you will add later. What you have offered, however, is an outline of the play; an indication of some of the potential dynamics between the actors, and a hint of some of the meaning that will emerge through your voice – the main character in the whole plot. I think that you offer enough here to illustrate how dramatic ordinary life can be. You also show how the simple business of organizing to help someone with a mental health problem can become hugely complex if we (therapists) forget what the experience of being helped might mean for the person. Finally, you show how we need also to try to see beyond the immediate therapeutic space, to catch a glimpse of the myriad of other meanings that the patient might bring along, which are connected to other would-be helpers, farther out or farther back on the stage.

The story of our therapy, which we shall develop in the subsequent chapters, is, therefore, no simple tale of one person trying to be of some help to another. Those other therapeutic relations framed the problem that you brought to me. You could hardly have been expected to accept me at 'face value', having had those other unsuccessful therapeutic relations who, in some respects, could have haunted our work. That our therapeutic relationship 'worked', without requiring a manifest exorcism of the other therapeutic players, is perhaps the most intriguing part of the whole story.

Your sketch for this 'play on your emotional life' also raises the critical issue about the fundamental nature of the therapeutic relationship, which we shall develop in other chapters. In many respects the counsellor and the analyst were unable to offer – or perhaps to sustain – the kind of relationship you needed. At least with the analyst, the relationship lacked some of the characteristics that you considered essential to 'a relationship'. The lay reader can be excused for assuming that a relationship cannot be one-way; it has to possess mutuality – one human engaging with another and *vice versa*. As Thomas Moore has eloquently written (Moore, 1994a):

> Every relationship, from the intense closeness of parents and child or partners in marriage, to the more distant connections with co-workers and business acquaintances, or even the driver of the bus we take daily to work, is an entanglement of souls. The gift in this entanglement is not only intimacy between persons, but also a revelation of soul itself, along with the invitation to enter more deeply into its mysteries. What better expresses the point of human life than engagement with this soul – with its manifest and hidden qualities, its mysterious alchemies and transformative pieties? If we can find the whole world in a grain of sand, we can also find the soul itself at the small point in life where destinies cross and hearts intermingle.

Regrettably – for me at least – much therapy has become dogged by the assumption that therapists can facilitate change in the patient without getting involved themselves. Crudely stated, this is like trying to rescue someone from drowning without getting wet in the process. True, it is possible to fish someone out of the water, but this is qualitatively very different from getting into the swim, with the person, and helping the person to safety (or salvation). The focus on the *mind* in therapy has also obscured the older fact that relationships are, as Moore wisely emphasized, about *soul-work* – repairing and potentially making whole again the souls of the two or more parties who are *relating*. This emphasis has long seemed true for my therapeutic work, even in the early stages when I know little of 'who' is the person who is the patient, and 'what' might be the full nature of the plot that will eventually unfold. This appreciation of the truly awesome nature of the life of another into which the therapist is privileged to step – preferably warily and carefully – renders the whole process a soulful experience.

You also introduce a critical subtext to the relationship; the issue of power. All relationships are powerful, but how 'power plays' occur within the whole play determines how the overarching power dynamic of the relationship operates and is experienced. Again, Thomas Moore draws attention to the nettle of power that needs grasping within relationships (Moore, 1994b):

> Every human relationship and interaction involves an exercise of power in which one person has some control over the other. We could make a microscopic analysis of a conversation between two people and graph the shifts in power. This power may be demonstrated as authority, strength of personality, emotion, articulateness, manipulation, guidance, knowledge, position – the possibilities are endless. The degree of dominance and submission also varies widely, so that in some interactions the imbalance may be very slight, while in others it is extreme.

Your sketch of the plot suggests how those different forms of power were used, by the therapists and by yourself, in this shifting ground called relating. The extent to which you were aware of your own power, if not also the extent to which your therapists knew theirs, is a critical part of the whole story, as you reflected later.

Entering therapy is an act of desperation. I had no idea what I was letting myself in for, and increased my anxiety greatly by imagining what might happen when I was alone with the therapist. What nightmares would I be tortured with? How much more would the traumas interfere with my ability to carry on my everyday life?

One of the reasons I chose originally to see a private counsellor was the flexibility to timetable sessions around my work schedule. Nobody, least of all my boss, needed to know of my arrangements. Work was very important to me, and I feared that if my superiors discovered I was in therapy, I would never again be trusted with the more taxing jobs. My career would take a dive, and my confidence and equanimity would be further eroded. Another plus for private counselling was the knowledge that there would be no permanent record of our meet-

ings which would follow me around in my medical file for the rest of my life.

Paradoxically, while the inability to carry on normal life was what sent me to the counsellor and to subsequent therapists, one of my primary considerations was that I should be able to carry on a normal life throughout the period of therapy. There were many times when I failed in that objective.

But how can we possibly know what we are in for when we present ourselves for therapy? So much depends on the quality of the relationship between the 'expert' helper and the one being helped. How difficult it is to suddenly open up to a complete stranger and tell him or her of feelings and experiences so private you can't even share them with your best friend. How difficult then to understand and accept the relationship on offer. How difficult to accept the soothing noises and professional patting. How confusing to be so intimate and dependent on someone who is not and probably never can be a real friend, yet for a significant period seems just that.

During the early sessions, the place of the meeting and the person being met crucially affect the progress of the therapeutic relationship. In those early days when my startle response was over-reacting, I experienced the telephone ringing as a very upsetting intrusion. In a busy hospital, where often the consulting room was literally a converted cupboard, I was traumatized by the voices of people passing constantly in the corridor outside or the voices of doctors and patients in adjoining rooms, and the incessant ringing of telephones. If I could hear them, they could hear me. Many times I left a session more anxious than when I arrived. You will recall that you held your clinic in a busy general hospital and had to battle against all these extra problems over and above my early communication difficulties. Somehow we managed, I think possibly because you didn't exacerbate the problem by chiding me for over-reacting to the outside stimuli – which I undoubtedly did. You would simply apologize, acknowledge the difficulty and attempt to move on, trying to help me 'wind down' in preparation for the real work of therapy.

Earlier, when I had begun to see the analyst, she too held her clinic in a busy general hospital, but soon suggested we meet at her office in a psychiatric hospital located in a pleasant rural setting a few miles out of town. The drive through country roads and into the tree-lined paths of the hospital was an excellent preparation for the work ahead. But in our early meetings I was frequently made anxious by the sound of gardeners working outside, or by staff and patients walking past the window of the ground-floor office. I asked the analyst if the curtains could be drawn, and when she told me to go ahead and close them myself I felt relieved that the world outside had been shut out, and a positive sense of having been able to take care of myself. Unfortunately, when I asked to close the curtains on our next meeting the request was refused, and I felt that I had been in the wrong to ask and my previous positive sense had been mis-

placed. My attempts to take care of myself and regain some of my control had backfired. This hampered the establishment of a therapeutic relationship, as I felt uncertain about suggesting things that might attract a 'black mark' against me.

The ambition for change

In the final analysis, your story is about ambition – the dream of wellness, of recovery, or at least the hope for diminution of distress. The 'point' of the therapeutic story is to reveal the different parts played by these three characters in your search for wholeness or emotional respite. Although you knew that this was to be your goal, at times the therapeutic process seemed to leave you even weaker than before – perhaps because you were opening yourself out to possibilities rather than defending yourself against the age-old possible threats. Early on in our relationship, you wrote:

This is too hard. If I did it properly it would make me hate myself and hate you. I don't want to do it. Anyway, I don't think I do things to make it OK most of the time. Most of the time it just is OK. But sometimes it's like I just give up. Whatever it is that makes me bounce out of bed in the morning, and get up everybody's nose because I grin too much in the lift at 9 am, just never shows up some days, and I don't know why. I sat and cried at the TV tonight but I don't know why. Sure, it was sad, but most days I wouldn't just sit and weep and not want to get up. It's not as easy to explain to myself as a definite problem that has a definite solution. Sometimes quite normal things just swamp me. I can't explain that. I can't tell you this is what I normally do to cope in this situation, because most of the time I don't think 'I am coping'. Most of the time I have no need to cope. I am happy with myself and my world. But what is it makes me walk into that (consulting) room and act like a normal human being and bounce out rejuvenated, ready to join in with the bustling outside, most of the time? Then, out of the blue, I'm terrified to leave that tiny room that's crushing in on me, and it is so unpleasant to be there. To open the door and look at all those faces rushing past, bustling about their business I feel detached from, is too terrifying – and I can't leave.

This early monologue revealed your fear and frustration with the whole process of reaching out to grasp that ambition of wholeness. So many questions, but no forthcoming answers.

As you looked back at that other Bobbie, who was beginning to reveal (again) the longing for wholeness, and experience the terror of 'breaking up', I wondered aloud what you made of all that, *now*? You turned to one of your favourite contemporary writers, William McIllvanney, who seemed to capture the gist of relationships that were focused on change and, by implication, were bound to be painful. His words seem like a fitting jumping off point for the rest of our reflections on relating (McIlvanney, 1998):

> Relationships that endured to the death could be impressive but they might merit more than sanctimonious paeans to the true nature of love. They might merit also questions. Constancy was a portmanteau, in which could sometimes be found, among other things, the senile decay of habit, the drug of comfort, the fear of change.

McIlvanney was talking about the most potent forms of human relating – that are found in everyday life, not in the orchestrated relatedness of therapy. However, his words light a moral signal for the therapist, who needs to be more than a constant in the maelstrom of mental distress. The kind of relationship that might help someone move beyond herself – rising up and stepping out of the corner into which she has retired – needs perhaps a more volatile kind of engagement. If the relationship is *for* any one thing, it is to breed curiosity (and hence questioning), and acknowledges that there are as many questions to be asked of the therapist as there are of the ambitious patient.

References

Driscoll, J. P. (1983). *Identity in Shakespearean Drama*, p. 182. Associated University Press.

Ferris, R. (1992). Hamlet and Romeo: Mark Rylance. In: *Shakespeare comes to Broadmoor* (M. Cox, ed.), p. 33. Jessica Kingsley.

McIlvanney, W. (1996). *The Kiln*, p. 267. Hodder and Stoughton.

Moore, T. (1994a). *Soul Mates: Honouring the Mysteries of Love and Relationship*, p. 259. Element.

Moore, T. (1994b). *Soul Mates: Honouring the Mysteries of Love and Relationship*, p. 216. Element.

3

Exploration

He felt again … the sadness of a failed relationship, not dulled by time but
sharpened by the greater understanding that time had given him. The deepest
grief wasn't in the mourning for what would no longer be but, given the
changed perception of your own experience, in the fear that it perhaps had
never been at all and you had dreamed it. For, if she had really been who you
thought she was, how was it possible for her to be who she later became? In
that despair could drown all hope, all belief in the value of your personal
experience. You might suspect that you would always live in an hallucination, had been doing that all your life.

McIlvanney (1998).

We in me – me in we

We are trapped, culturally if not also psychologically, into believing that
therapy is a curative or a restorative process. Therapy is something that
the therapist dispenses, even when he is just using himself to do the necessary giving – *the therapeutic use of self.* Such assumptions are clearly
important, for without such a moral basis for the practice of therapy the
whole activity might be viewed as far too uncertain, completely beyond
control, and requiring no specific responsibility or accountability on the
therapist's part. However, just because the therapist has *some* responsibilities and is accountable for his actions does not mean that he is
responsible for the essence of the therapeutic process itself. Indeed, by
taking care of his own input and avoiding overestimating the extent or
power of his influence over the proceedings, the therapist may eventually
reach an understanding of what is going on, what might need to be done,
and whether or not he has the capacity to do this. Throughout the whole

encounter, in addition to keeping one eye (and ear) on the patient, the therapist needs to keep an eye on himself, watching and listening to what is happening *to* him, as well as *through* him. As we begin to talk about the importance of the exploration of the patient's lifeworld, it is important to acknowledge that such self-awareness on the part of the therapist is, arguably, just as important. Indeed, the two parties who come together to construct the therapeutic conversation are watching one another, watching themselves, watching the other.

Exploring through metaphor

Many relationships ultimately become difficult to fathom, becoming gummed up, so to speak, by the sticky web which goes to make up those relations in the first place. The mixing of metaphors doesn't entirely escape me here. Indeed, mixing metaphors when trying to talk of inter-personal *relations* or therapist–patient *relationships* is almost like mixing colours on our narrative palette. The riches of human relatedness demands metaphors. Indeed, we may only begin to understand what we 'know' in our hearts of our experience of our relationships through use of such metaphors. For what part of ourselves is relating, in what partic-ular way, to which part of some other person, and what – if anything – is cementing, or supporting, or helping such a relation between two quite different persons, from two very different worlds of experience? I make a big assumption here – that the world of personal experience is a unique world. If there can be an answer to the question I pose, it can hardly be an easy one – at least not unless we grossly oversimplify it by reducing it (metaphorically) to some hypothetical parts, functions, processes or elements.

Such is the transparent reliance on metaphor in ordinary everyday dis-course that we deceive ourselves into believing that we know what *exactly* we are talking about, when – as Aristotle astutely observed – metaphor is no more or less than giving a name to one thing that belongs to something else[1]. The idea of one person developing, or being involved in, or enjoying, or being affected by ' a relationship' involving another, is a complex idea, to say the least. To some extent that complexity is tied up (metaphorically) in the language we use to express what we know – epistemologically – of the relationship: how it feels, what we think about, when we reflect on ourselves and the self that is the 'other'. The inherent complexity of the relations between one person and another become writ large when we turn our attention to even closer forms of human related-ness: our relations with ourselves; when we begin to consider who might be the 'I' who is 'me'?

---

[1]In all our talk about mental illness and health, the sagest contemporary appreciation of the central role of metaphor is to be found in the writings of Thomas Szasz (see Szasz, 1990).

William McIlvanney aptly described the sheer complexity of the relationship riddle in the opening to this chapter. His character laments the loss of something within his 'failed relationship' – a thing which he has turned, unwittingly, into an object of loss. He considers how the object of his sadness, the other half of his 'failed relationship', might not have been a constant at all, but might have been, essentially, a moving, changing, shifting 'thing'. In so doing, he feels the fear many of us feel when we confront the absolute uncertainty of everyday life. Then, like McIlvanney's character, we doubt the experience, which has long been the mainstay of our very 'being' – the thing that has, moment by moment, advised us that we are 'being'. And perhaps we too begin to wonder if life is any more than a dream, if not a mere hallucination.

Not all people who enter or graduate from therapy have such complex human riddles anywhere near the top of their therapeutic agenda. However, when the patient eventually looks back, metaphorically, down all the days that serve as the timeframe for the therapeutic process, she may begin to appreciate the extent to which her very 'self' might have been no more than an idea framed in words. Moreover, she may appreciate further the extent to which that verbalized 'self' is an idea subject to fickle shifts of emphasis, overstatement and paraphrasing. Life may be neither dream nor hallucination, but its description relies heavily on the same language and grammar of experience necessary to account for dreams and hallucinations. Ironically, however, our waking selves may be less sensitive (more asleep) to the metaphorical messages that we appreciate intuitively in dreams, but blinker (paradoxically) in the illumination of the mind by day.

You appeared to appreciate the need to frame your experiences of distress and therapy in metaphorical if not overtly symbolic terms when you first noted that what had 'happened to you' was that, over time, you had 'lost your nerve for living'.

I remember meeting a survivor of the Piper Alpha disaster many months after he had been rescued from the inferno. He told me he could not bear the telephone ringing, which he experienced as the outside world encroaching on him. He refused to leave the cocoon of his own home. He had been a scaffolder, and spoke with a passion about his work high up on the steel climbing frames of building sites. He was a king in that domain. But after the Alpha disaster he lost his nerve, said he'd probably forget where he was if he ever went up high again, said he'd just walk off the end in a daydream. But it wasn't just the scaffolding he was scared of. He had lost his nerve for living.

On each occasion I began a new therapeutic relationship, I too had lost my nerve for living. I was looking for someone to grab me before I walked off the end. A person in this state is barely able to make a decision, certainly not one so complex as the choice of an appropriate therapist. People in a distressed state haven't the skills to make such an important judgement, but in that respect are little different from people of sound mind. Laymen simply don't have sufficient knowledge of the speciality. I know nothing about cars. If I have a problem with my vehicle, I take it to a garage and trust I will get expert help. There are good garages and bad garages, and sometimes we can't tell the difference until the damage has been done. Therapists are no different from car mechanics. Something needs to be sorted. We know that. What we don't know is how to sort it.

Of course, we know what to call such experiences – *post-traumatic stress disorder.* Somehow, this technical label seems to confer little more human understanding than having 'lost one's nerve for living'. Indeed, by turning the experience into a 'thing', we may have lost some appreciation of what is going on *within* the experience, what helps to create and maintain the 'thing'. I think that you know, in the scary chambers of your heart, what I mean.

(Re)discovering the I and me in we

I make no apologies for problematizing[2] the relations that, linguistically, appear to develop when one person (the therapist) meets another (the patient). For, at the same time, there appears to be no less a complex set of ongoings when the patient *reflects* on herself. However, putting such complexities to one side – if that is possible – we might ask, what might be the *essence* of the therapeutic process? What *happens*, that is not the direct result of the therapist's input? If this essential element is not the result of the therapist's influence, then how does it come about, and who *is* bringing this to fruition?

To answer such technically simple yet humanly profound questions, we need to retrace our steps, asking ourselves what the whole business of therapy might be 'about'. What is the proper focus of the therapeutic endeavour? We need to ask these banal yet critical questions if we are even to begin to appreciate what we believe happens in therapy.

Therapy is always about exploration and discovery, but I didn't realize that until much later in the whole process. When I read through my journal again, about a year later, I realized that problems I had been chewing over in the journal were still with me, still very much on the agenda. I think the difference now is that when you are in therapy – at least at the start – the first thing you have to learn is to identify the prob-

---

[2]Although this introduction to the processes and parameters of 'the relationship' may be interpreted from a Sullivanian, or a structuralist, perspective, my allusions to the central function of metaphor in most verbal communications about such human communications reveals my leanings towards a post-structuralist analysis of the 'truth' of such human dealings (Derrida, 1976; Evans, 1996).

lems. Once you are able to do that, much later, you can learn how to work out practical ways of resolving those problems: solutions to problems and ways of living with things that simply can't be solved.

That's the difference that is most obvious, looking at the journal from where I stand now. Back then, when I was writing it, I had only just started formulating the idea that I had a problem – for example, with my friend Jennifer. Now I can trace the evolution of that particular problem, and I feel quite confident about my solution. Back then, on the page of the journal, I could never have contemplated just walking away from the relationship. However, that is exactly what I had to do. Indeed, that is what, eventually, I did – exactly. I now feel so much stronger for having done that. I've done it all by myself.

Although the subject matter of therapy is obviously talk – stories and the whole narrative that is taking shape – its felt *meaning is more obvious, yet at the same time more subtle. Therapy comes to be about the possibilities for what can be done in everyday life, as well as ways around frustrations: ways of dealing with, in Shakespeare's fine phrase,* the slings and arrows of outrageous fortune. *Although this is a challenge that most people have to face at some time, for the person in therapy it appears to represent a particular set of challenges. If therapy is about exploring and discovering, I would say it involves meeting Mistress Uncertainty with your head up.*

It seems ironic that, at the end of the second millennium, having made so much technological progress, humanity should still be struggling with Mistress Uncertainty. Yet despite the adolescent strivings of our post-modern society, which often tries to turn life into commerce, complete with its assurances as to quality and standards, life follows its own often inscrutable rhythm. As Alan Watts noted (Watts, 1997):

> the life that we live is a contradiction and a conflict ... to strive for pleasure to the exclusion of pain is, in effect, to strive for the loss of consciousness. Because such a loss is in principle the same as death, this means that the more we struggle for life (pleasure) the more we are actually killing what we love.

Yet for many people such a goal – control over *all* life circumstances – holds great attraction, perhaps the same attraction that Midas first saw in the golden touch. Confronting life, walking away from people and things, finding that some things change and others appear to remain the same whatever we try to do, are the only facts of which we can be certain. The realization of such an ephemeral understanding of the innate fickleness of life confers what Watts called '*the wisdom of insecurity*' (Watts, 1997). Alternatively, our struggles to impose order on an unruly human universe lead at first to tears of frustration and disappointment, and ultimately – at least for Watts – to the death of the spirit:

It is understandable that we should sometimes ask ... whether 'the game is worth the candle', and whether it might be better to turn the course of evolution in the only other possible direction – backwards, to the relative peace of the animal, the vegetable and the mineral.

Something of this kind is often attempted. There is the woman who, having suffered some deep emotional injury, vows never to let another man play on her feelings, assuming the role of the hard and bitter spinster. Almost more common is the sensitive boy who learns in school to encrust himself for life in the shell of the 'tough guy' attitude. As an adult he plays, in self defence, the role of the Philistine, to whom all intellectual and emotional culture is womanish and 'sissy'. Carried to its final extreme, the logical end of this type of reaction to life is suicide. The hard-bitten kind of person is always, as it were, a partial suicide; some of himself is already dead.

Real everyday living

When I was in therapy, there was never a point when I geared myself up and said, 'I wonder what we'll explore today?'. However, there were times during those sessions, and more often outwith the sessions when I was alone, that I would surprise myself. Looking back, it was in those moments that I made real discoveries. After I surprised myself, I felt refreshed. I had learned something important and could move on more confidently.

Often the discoveries were very simple, like when I discovered the joy of creativity in making soup. As a committed, fully paid-up member of the microwave generation, I came late to the realization that spending three hours making soup from scratch offered a satisfaction that outstrips the ritual opening of tins of condensed liquid.

Maybe there are some parallels with therapy there. Maybe dealing with the raw materials of life is akin to washing, scraping and chopping carrots. Maybe enlightenment really is to be found in peeling the potatoes, rather than meditating on the Buddha. It is just such illustrations of the everyday magic of experience that suggest the spiritual underbelly of our lives. The excesses of the New Age movement and the confused relationship with religion have led many to reject the notion of any such spiritual core to our lives. Your example suggests the possibilities for exploring the spiritual in everyday life in very small ways, revealing in the process something of the meaning of such (extra)ordinary experience.

What is explored in therapy is, I imagine, much the same for everybody. At the root of all our discussions is an exploration of what is important to us; how we want to live our lives, and how we go about achieving that goal. Of course, what we decide is important, and how we put our plans into action will be different for everyone, but the aim remains much the same for all of us.

One of the things that the therapist might explore is *how* the patient *is:* what is happening for her at any given moment, and what she is doing, actively, as part of that process of being. I am sure that my curious enquiries must often have sounded irritatingly naïve – perhaps even *faux-naif.* When you would begin to describe an episode in your life, my enquiries sought to reveal more of the events on various levels, but also to reveal how these events were not truly episodes at all but flowed into and through the succeeding 'episodes' in your life:

- Tell me more!
- And what was that like?
- And how did you feel?
- And what happened next?

These questions assumed that the narrative that flowed from your pen into your journal was part of a much bigger 'flow' of experience. One might describe it as an inexhaustible flow of experience that continually generated and regenerated itself through the living of your life and your reflections on living. My curiosity was focused less on the details of *what* had happened, but on the processes that had somehow brought these 'happenings' into your awareness. And so I often asked the grossly naïve but highly exploratory question – 'how *did* you *do* that?'.

In the early sessions, when you were experiencing great distress or reflecting on how distress had haunted you down many of the days of your life, I asked about how you *had* coped with these experiences, indeed what you *did* now to cope. Many therapists would describe this as a manipulative question. You are talking about the 'failure to cope' that had brought you into contact with three previous therapists, and I appear to ignore this state of affairs and ask how you *do* cope. My assumption – or rather presumption – was justified since, like so many other people who had sat in the patient's chair and recounted the various tragic, scary and damaging events of their experience, clearly you could have been in much more dire straits. I was curious to know *what* had kept you from rattling down further, from being even more damaged by your life experience. The question must, at times, have seemed like a daft one.

I think the reason I didn't want to do this, or rather that it was difficult to think about, was that I was going at the question from a different angle from you. You asked, what do I do to cope? But I'm not aware of coping, only when I don't cope. I start to think about your question, then shutdown because inevitably I get snarled up in what was upsetting me when

I didn't cope rather than thinking about what I might have done to prevent throwing a wobbler.

Anyway, while I was having a cupboard clearout the other day I came across a collection of cuttings about a good friend of mine who was charged under the Official Secrets Act in 1982. It made me think about all the bad things that happened that year, and the fact I didn't lose the place. I had to be doing something right then, because 1982 definitely qualifies as the year the greatest number of bad things happened to me.

In March 1982 I wanted to go to London and visit my best friend from school. I go down to see her regularly, but I knew that year she didn't want to see me and kept putting me off. I didn't know what I'd done wrong, but I got the message I wasn't welcome. It turned out she was having a baby in April and she hadn't told anyone at home, including her mum and dad. She just took leave from work and took care of the situation all alone until she had the baby, when it was taken away for adoption.

Lesley didn't tell me about all that until the October of that year. We had had a death in the family a couple of months earlier[3], and she had written me a really nice letter (I still have all those letters, and that's one of the things I do when I am feeling abandoned and sorry for myself – read the wee notes from all my closest friends, which are all pretty short but say a lot). Anyway, Lesley invited me down to London in the October, and she was talking about the person we lost, then she pulled out this wee wallet of photos and told me it was her baby she gave away when she was three days old. I just didn't know what to do for her, but in the end I decided she just needed me to know, not to do or say anything in particular. However, she was hurting bad.

The other ongoing situation that year was Andrea being charged under the Official Secrets Act. I owe her a lot, because it was she who persuaded me to abandon University. It was the best thing I ever did, because I made my mind up to go for what I really wanted – which was to write – and life just took off from there. The trouble was, when Andrea got into difficulties I was nowhere for her. She had left her lecturing job and gone abroad to work. (With hindsight I think the reason she was so keen for me abandon University and make major life changes was because she was trying to make a similar commitment herself!)

Anyway, she left her job and became a diplomat, but in 1982 she was charged with passing classified information. It was in all the nationals, but reporting restrictions were never lifted. Anyway, when I saw the stories, knowing Andrea I knew there would be a man in it somewhere and the 'secrets' pillow talk. I was right, but her 'brilliant' career was ruined and I just watched as the worst excesses of journalism got to work. The tabloids dredged up ancient photos of her from home, and grabbed any comment they could from unnamed acquaintances. I never

---

[3] I don't say at this point that the death is that of my brother.

got in touch with her (well, not until much later when it had all publicly blown over), and I never told anyone I had recent photos, could do a proper biography, and had names and 'phone numbers of real friends. To me I could see I had a great story, but I never, ever would have done that to Andrea.

I got a letter from her this week saying she has got a new job as a senior administrative assistant in the department of law and administration in a local council – 'whatever that means', she says. It means she will be back in court arguing over licensing applications, etc. Even ten years on, I think it will take some doing, walking back into a court again.

Anyway, all this was by way of background to show why 1982 was a pretty tough year, but I never cracked. Thinking now why that might have been, I think it is very simple. All that year, the person who died[4] had been training me to run my first marathon. I wanted us to run together, but he said that there was no way he would be able to keep up all the training, but he would stand at the finish holding my tracksuit and acting as my number one fan! Of course he wasn't there in the end, but I felt I had to keep up the training and reach the goal. My days all had a structure of running and making sure I ate properly. I was running two hours at a time and, if I went out in the morning before a late shift, it would make me 'high' for the rest of the day. I had no bad energy that burst out unexpectedly at inappropriate times. Anyway, maybe it seems too simplistic an answer to you, but I really think, to keep on an even keel, I need regular physical exercise. Anyway, I've decided to take up running again – not so it's a chore I have to do every day and something I've got to be the very best I can possibly be at, because that starts up bad feelings too, but just as a way of expending dangerous energy.

The enduring quality of water

It was obvious that I needed to explore some of the darker corners of your life. If I hadn't done that then you might have felt cheated, since this is – by general consensus – the whole 'point' of therapy; to shine light into the darker recesses of past experience. However, without knowing how disastrous some of those past 'exploratory' attempts had been for you, I chose to focus on what was 'working' for you in your life and the living of it. I chose to focus on exploring some of the corners of your experience that were lit, however dimly. I presumed that these light spots existed, and I wanted to draw them into your awareness. When you looked back on the whole experience of the therapeutic process, you seemed to appreciate the intuitive timing of those particular explorations.

---

[4]My brother.

Exploration and discovery begins very tentatively. We do not trust our-selves. We are afraid of what we will see when we look closely at our-selves. We are certainly afraid of others and, looking back through my diaries and letters, I can see clearly how I held you, initially, at arm's length. I was chewing over very important things for me. Even though I was addressing you (the therapist), the text reads like a private conver-sation, as I was (clearly) not giving enough information – for example, when I was talking about my dead brother and I referred to 'someone I used to know'. This reference was a perfectly truthful description, but for you it must have been like wading through treacle, trying to understand what I was talking about.

The early diaries and letters contrast sharply with the straightforward familiarity of the later texts. However, it was only in looking back and re-reading the texts that I became aware of just how sharp the contrast was. I was able to discover again just how vital to the process of healing is the relationship that is forged between the therapist and the patient, and how critical this is to the eventual breaking away.

In re-reading the texts, I was able to discover again that we kept on exploring and discovering. The constructions of meaning I gave to events and situations at the start of therapy were very different by the end. Indeed, they are different again as I look back now. What we learn and the meaning we give to things is fluid. The construction I have put on my experiences is in a continual state of flux. That appreciation is no longer threatening; it is (now) exciting. It is what enables us to jump out of bed in the morning and wonder what the day might hold. We are hopeful, not cowed.

As I look at this last paragraph, I notice that I have slipped into using 'we' and 'us'. That was not conscious, but I realize that when we are ill we are obsessed with ourselves and our crippling fears. When we are well, we feel connected to everyone else. We realize that the people we meet in the street, at work and in the supermarket all have problems. We are no longer special because we are suffering a bit. Eventually we are liberated by this knowledge.

The heart-felt wisdom of these few lines lies, in my humble view, in the appreciation of the fluidity of experience. I have lived most of my life near water. Late in life I realized that this might not have been entirely accidental. I might have been drawn to live and spend time near water, because of traumatic early childhood experiences involving water, or perhaps simply because I was born under a water star-sign. Humankind has fostered a deep but less than honest relationship with the concept of permanence. Today in particular we contemplate the promise that genetic manipulation might allow us to live for ever. Like children who don't want the party to end, such a contrived immortality would save us the grief of living with dying. But would such immortality promise us hap-piness, or fulfilment, or any of the other simple human achievements that 'we' have sought down the ages? I think not. The promise that we need not address the ultimate point of life (death) seems to be a curious promise indeed.

We learn early in life that the earth is solid. Maybe that is why we develop the tendency to become hard-nosed materialists. However, the solidity of our experience belies its impermanence, and disguises the quantum reality that, ultimately, sheer nothingness lies at the heart of all that we assume to be solid. I should say that I *believe* what the physicists say, rather than understand it. I'm not sure what, exactly, all the implications of quantum reality means in physical terms.

However, even staying with the surface reality, I *know* – experientially – that my everyday experience is characterized by fluidity, by flux, by impermanence, and that the idea that 'I' am in any way stable, established or grounded is a construction that I put on my experience of myself. As you reflected on your experiences – ultimately committing them to paper and, at another remove, reading what you had written – you developed a deep appreciation of the consistency of impermanence; the trustworthiness of the fickle state of your being in the world. Perhaps perversely, I find something remarkably reassuring in the idea of a fickle, unpredictable universe of experience.

Here seems a good point to address the virtue of reflection and the value of committing such reflections to paper. Therapy may have given you some boundaries, a specific context or a frame of reference for your experience. However, we should not lose sight of what lay within – the experience of experience itself. If you were exploring any one thing, it was that experience of experience.

Gerhard Durlacher disappeared into Auschwitz-Birkenau in 1944, still a boy, but of course a Jewish boy. He was one of the fortunate few to survive the experience and, after the war in Holland, he studied and eventually became a sociology professor. The remarkable feature of his story (Durlacher, 1998) was that he never talked about any of his memories to his wife or children until the last ten years of his life. When his physical illnesses became so unmanageably chronic, his doctor recognized that his 'illness' might not lie in his body after all, but in his mind and the traumas of those dark childhood days. Once Durlacher had been 'opened up' by a psychiatrist who specialized in treating victims of the Holocaust, using LSD, he began to develop a fascination for his lost past. He had spent years keeping his past under wraps, telling himself that 'he needed to stamp on it, to quench it like a volcano'. Now he realized the need to explore, through reflection, his experience of those awful experiences. He needed to look into the mirror of his soul.

We would hope that Gerhard's story and the eventual 'telling' of it would have a happy ending; complete with the healing of his old wounds and the conferment of some special blessing on his wife and, by now, grown up daughters. Sadly, this was not to be. His wife could not cope with the demands of trying to help Gerhard with his gruesome work.

Trying to type up his tapes reduced her to helpless fits of tears. His eldest daughter felt suffocated by the whole process and left home, only later revealing how she had accepted some of her father's suffering in the development of her anorexia.

The sadness felt and expressed by the daughters – that they should not have had to learn of their father's distress in this way, from a book – will strike a chord with many people. How many of us really *know* our parents, far less the other lives that float past us on the river of life? For Gerhard, the process ended in him reaching a conclusion that was the opposite of what he had first hoped for. The confrontation of all the fears and horrors of his childhood spawned six books in which he recorded many of those experiences and his efforts to make sense of them. He had hoped that, as a sociologist, he would find an explanation for it all, and for his survival in particular. However, he eventually concluded that there was no explanation. He could not say *why* he had survived, only *how* it is to survive.

As I sit now, reading his words, I reflect on the similarities with your story (however different) and all the stories of those who confront the demons of their past, which appear to inhabit them rather than simply haunt them. I am struck by the fact that it is *how* anyone survives at all that is the explanation we really seek. The exploration of experience does not seek to explain away the experience. The exploration of experience does not necessarily lead to territorial control over that which has been explored, as if we were exploring and discovering new land. For the land-scape is not in any way new – it is merely our back pages or, to continue the water metaphor, the backwaters of experience, some of the farther reaches of our humanity. As we give the power of our historic nightmares the form of words, we may not always exorcize that awful power. However, by exorcizing it in language we reform it, and the story becomes apparent – part of the tangled yarn that is the web of life.

Mountain reflected in a pool

There is a common assumption that somehow, through exploration and reflection, we can 'get to the bottom' of things in our lives. However hard we engage with our experience, we cannot prevent the addition of new layers of appreciation and meaning. The simple act of looking at our reflection produces another layer of meaning. Such is the simple law of human dynamics – through looking, everything changes and, in a sense, also remains the same.

I hope you don't mind me writing to you, but I haven't finished talking to you yet and the next appointment seems a long way away. I wouldn't like to have all this stuff buzzing about in my head for two whole weeks.

Last night I was lying chewing over what we'd been saying to each other and finding some things I wish I had said but didn't. (That said, there was probably plenty I did say that I shouldn't have.) I'm sorry I was so awkward. I don't mean to be difficult, but there seems to be a huge gulf between knowing (or thinking I know) what to do and actually going ahead and getting stuck in.

I was chewing over your question about how far up the mountain did I think I was. I know it must seem a very straightforward question to you, but I really wasn't dodging you when I said I couldn't answer. It was a really difficult question for me.

This is my attempt to answer it, now I've had a chance to think about it. I'm sure I told you that the last time I saw the analyst I felt that I was only just beginning. In one way that seems daft, because I can remember vividly the date of my first appointment. But knowing that still doesn't take away the feeling that I am just at the beginning in some ways.

When you ask me to think about the problem that brought me for help, that's when I feel I haven't got anywhere, because I haven't done anything to address that problem or change how I feel about it.

However, when I think back to the start of last summer, the main problem had been overtaken. I had stopped being able to function at the simplest level. The crisis didn't occur when I was sitting in court listening to the story of a child abuser; it happened when I was at a routine meeting. I felt totally swamped, unable to do the job adequately, when I should've been able to do it standing on my head with my hands tied behind my back. Instead, I just started to shake and couldn't stop.

There were other ordinary things I couldn't do at that time. I would suddenly get the feeling I couldn't be alone, and would take myself off to friends unannounced. Once there, I would just as suddenly feel unsettled being there, and be unable to stay. That doesn't happen any more.

Also, I have started to read for pleasure again. I am really grateful to have that back. This time last year I couldn't concentrate on a novel, and would read the same page over and over again and still not know what I had read. Eventually I just gave up reading everything but the local newspaper, and I was even paranoid about that.

The other thing that is different is my trick of jumping ten feet in the air when a 'phone rings, a doorbell goes or there is any sudden noise. Lots of people have commented on the absence of this, though that I know is down to the pills I still have to take every day.

Anyway, these are just examples to show that there has been demonstrable progress. Now if we go back to your mountain image, my answer is that I have made progress but I still feel I am just beginning. To put it in mountain terms, every time I get to the top of the mountain, I've only really got up onto a ridge and another summit has loomed up ahead of me and I know there's another big climb ahead. I think that's my answer to your question anyway. I couldn't answer at the time, because I didn't want to make you think you'd been completely wasting your time if I'd said I was still at the foot of the mountain. Now I realize that we have just *been finding our way through the foothills before we go on for the main assault. Does that make sense to you?*

The other thing I am aware of is how a climber has to have complete faith in his climbing partner and his equipment. His personal safety depends on that. This is certainly the case with us; however, it is what is making me most afraid just now. I am aware I am taking more risks with you, going into dangerous territory and hoping we will stay safe.

What makes it very hard is that I feel like I have been here before and I know there's a big drop when your partner lets go of the rope. So I get scared when I hear things and feel things (even good things). It's hard for me to have any faith in my own judgement.

On the other hand, I don't want to spend my life wandering about the foothills. I want to keep going on and up, but I know that mountaineering is not a solo sport and I have still got the hope I will get it right this time and not fall off the end of the rope or make you untie the safety knots. Sometime you will stay behind in basecamp and I'll head on up to the top and raise the Lion Rampant!

These reflections on the therapeutic climb begin to suggest the true challenges that are emerging for you, or that you glimpse some way off in the distance. They also suggest the importance of exploring with a partner, if not as part of a team. However, despite the value of collegiality, as Walt Whitman (1965) vigorously said:

NOT I – NOT ANYONE else, can travel that road for you. You must travel it for yourself.

And, in the spirit of stepping out on your own road, you made this entry.

Well, now I've done something either very brave or very stupid. I've had a letter I got in a Christmas card sitting around here for ages. It's from a girl I used to know, inviting me to come and visit her and her young family. I haven't seen her for years. In fact, I haven't seen her since she was a schoolgirl. She was my late brother's girlfriend. I always think you shouldn't go back, but I can't resist it. She describes her domestic bliss with two toddlers, and it sounds just like I imagined she'd end up all those years ago. That will be nice to see, but I just wonder if it will point up the contrast between the reality and the imagined for the person we both used to know. I think that's why I'm going; to see if I can deal with that, like a test for myself. Even if I enjoy my day out, I might never go again. Maybe letting go is not going at all, but at the moment I feel I haven't really let go unless I can face up to the past (that is, go and visit Karen) but not NEED to go again. That is, I want to know I'm not afraid to go, that I can 'cope' with that situation if I choose to. I am not simply avoiding the situation. But if you ask me what practical things I can do to cope in the situation, I can't tell you. I just have to have faith that I will.

Of course, finding your own faith may have been the true endpoint of all your explorations. However, given all your concerns about how far you might have travelled, and to what extent you were any way past your starting point, T. S. Eliot's observation seems apposite (Eliot, 1942):

> What we call the beginning is often the end
> And to make an end is to make a beginning
> The end is where we start from.

If the journey out appeared to run into the journey back, maybe that was simply because the act of journeying was the real event, rather than any discoveries made along the way. Again, Eliot distils the essence of that journey which all of us need to take:

> We shall not cease from exploration
> And the end of all our exploring
> Will be to arrive where we started
> And to know the place for the first time.

References

Derrida, J. (1976). *De la grammatologie* (translated by G. Chakravorty). John Hopkins University Press.

Durlacher, G. (1988). *The Search*. Serpent's Tail.

Eliot, T. S. (1979). *Little Gidding. Four Quartets*. Faber and Faber.

Evans, F. B. (1996). *Harry Stack Sullivan: Interpersonal Theory and Psychotherapy*. Routledge.

McIlvanney, W. (1996). *The Kiln*, p. 165. Hodder and Stoughton.

Szasz, T. *Insanity: The Idea and its Consequences*, pp. 135–69. John Wiley and Sons.

Watts, A. (1997). *The Wisdom of Insecurity: A Message for an Age of Anxiety*, p. 29. Rider.

Whitman, W. (1965). *Leaves of Grass*, p. 79. Airmont Publishing Company Inc.

4

Words – the bridge between two worlds

To the dispassionate onlooker therapy is just two people talking – and they are right.

Language, experience and power

Therapy is an educational experience for both therapist and patient. I recognize that I enter the therapeutic arena knowing virtually nothing of the *person* who is the patient. If fortunate, I might gain something of an education as to the true human standing of the patient by the close of our relationship. Ultimately, however, I often have to settle for knowing little of any real consequence about this unique human specimen.

That said, uniqueness is not exactly prized in the circles that confine the helping arts. Instead, there is a concern to label and classify the person's experience, demystifying it by likening it to the experience of others. 'Gee,' the person-cum-patient might well say, 'I thought I was going crazy, then I found out it was *only* schizophrenia!' (or any one of several other so-called 'conditions'). Ironically, we are all more like one another than different or, as Harry Stack Sullivan wisely observed, 'we are all more simply human than otherwise'. On that occasion, Sullivan was talking about people trapped in psychotic states (Sullivan, 1953). He recognized that such people (as opposed to objectified patients) were not having an alien experience, but were offering him an opportunity to examine the range of his own experience of selfhood, the illusory boundaries of his own notions of sanity. Paradoxically, the therapists' efforts to re-define the unique experiences of people when they are in one state of 'patienthood' or another, sets them apart from so-called normals, who preciously guard the differences between themselves and the neurotics, obsessionals or those who are just plain 'mad'. I suppose that is the enduring attraction of psychiatric labels to define *and* explain our human distress – they offer us the illusion that there remains nothing fundamentally wrong with 'us', but that somehow some abstract psychiatric avenger, who robs us of the patina of sanity, has assailed the 'us' in 'we'.

I believed that if I could remain sufficiently open to the experience I might learn something of value about you, and perhaps much about myself. The nature of the therapeutic contract is such that I need to work very hard not to learn something about both of us. The therapeutic contract usually demands that patients talk and therapists listen. There is an expectation that the patient will tell her story, or as much of it as she is able, but the therapist need offer as little of himself and his story as he wishes. As you note in later chapters, my approach to the therapeutic contract was a little unconventional, not least to the extent that I too was keen to talk, and in so doing reveal something of myself. However, even under such unconventional conditions our therapeutic relationship remained a lopsided arrangement, and with that came responsibility, which we shall address in later chapters. Here we focus on some aspects of your 'story' and the whole 'storying' process, especially on how the abstract dimensions of experience found some shape through the limitations of words (De Shazer, 1991).

Although most forms of psychotherapy acknowledge the central importance of the unique experience of the patient, the influence of our technological society has heightened the demands to place psychotherapy on a more scientific footing[1]. However, such ambition risks losing sight of the person, who may become occluded by the construction of the patient required of such a scientific endeavour. If a human science of psychotherapy is possible, perhaps it will be a development of the patient's personal science. I have little idea of what exactly various patients with whom I have worked have experienced. I have, however, shared by mutual agreement my experience of their reflections on their personal science. Many of them, in turn, presumably had a reciprocal sharing of *my* experience of *their* experience. The inherent complexity of those interactions is difficult to get one's tongue around. The linguistic knots betray the truth of Wittgenstein's assertion that language is the only reality. As he observed (Wittgenstein, 1965):

> … let's not forget that a word hasn't got a meaning given to it, as it were, by a power independent of us, so that there could be a kind of scientific investigation into what the word really means. A word has the meaning someone has given to it.

---

[1]This is not really a new phenomenon, since Freud (1924) first framed this ambition, noting that he 'always felt it a gross injustice that people have refused to treat psychoanalysis like any other science' (see Gay, 1995).

Bakhtin had earlier made a similar observation that was very important for the business of therapy. In Bakhtin's view, when people are conversing, complete versions of reality are not being passed back and forth, rather (Todorov, 1984):

> no utterance in general can be attributed to the speaker exclusively; it is the product of the interaction ... and, broadly speaking, the product of the whole complex social situation in which it has occurred.

Of course, we all believe that 'we' are doing the main pushing or pulling of our own reality, prodding and kneading it into shape. This suggests something of our relationship with language. The language that defines my experience also serves as the boundary for my knowledge of myself and of others. Language, as Peplau noted, influences thought; thought then influences action; and thought and action together evoke feelings in relation to situations or contexts (Peplau, 1969). Here, Peplau was talking of the power of language in any situation. The language used in professional helping has an even more specialized and powerful function. The language of psychotherapy, largely because of its association with medicine, has acquired a disempowering function. As Illich (1976) noted, since language was taken over by doctors:

> the sick person is deprived of meaningful words for his anguish, which is further increased by linguistic mystification.

Although we have been aware for almost fifty years of how language may be manipulated to put distance and boundaries between patient and professional (Whorf, 1956), the dialogue between patient and professional often continues to be more tortuous than, arguably, is necessary. However, by artificially keeping the patient at a distance the tortured prose of psychobabble helps to protect the world of the therapist – even if the protection that language offers is illusory. Regrettably even this is no longer true, as many patients have begun to learn the language of therapy (and all other forms of psychobabble), perhaps in a misguided attempt to regain some control over their experience.

Unfolding awareness

Therapy began to work for me when I was able to find the words to tell my stories, when I began to feel that I was not only able to explain to myself the sadness, fears and failures of my life but that I was able to share that unfolding awareness in a meaningful way with my therapist.

Of course, it could be asked, what else could therapy involve if not the development of awareness and the deeper appreciation of meaning, not

to mention a little sharing? However, the sheer simplicity of that observation betrays its importance. People come to therapy wishing to put
down or otherwise rid themselves of some weight they are carrying. Or
they come because someone else thinks they need some of that special
unburdening. Either way, the assumption is that the therapist will
somehow *do* the unburdening, releasing the patient from her emotional
chains. In truth, the patient does the very hard work that is involved in
unfolding awareness and revealing meaning.

It becomes such hard work for the simple reason that the patient, and
especially those around her – family and friends, and everyone else who
would act in her best interests – believe that unburdening *must* involve
hard work. I must confess that often I have felt like some life tourist,
standing idly by as someone in the thick of life digs vigorously in the
noonday sun, trying to reveal that elusive meaning. And as I listen to my
own plaintive voice, I seem to be saying little more than: 'How are you
doing? Found anything of interest?' I certainly often felt that way as I
watched you labour to reach that point of 'meaningful communication'
which came to mean so much to you.

I hadn't really thought about my work in such terms before, but now I
wonder how much this notion of 'idling' while others 'labour' stems from
my own conflicts over my working class roots. I broke with the tradition
of my forefathers, and instead of making something within time –
digging a ditch, building a house – my labour involves only plays on
words. Although my forefathers might wonder when I was going to begin
to work at all, my conflict lies in trying to make sure that I don't work
too hard. However much I might *want* to see you make progress, this
would be no more than vain ambition on my part. Joseph Campbell recognized this need to keep clear of other people's experience lest we contaminate it with our own:

> What each must seek in his life never was on land or sea. It is something
> out of his own unique potentiality for experience, something that never has
> been and never could have been experienced by anyone else. (Boldt, 1997)

The benefit of therapeutic idleness is that in time the patient comes to
much the same kind of realization as you did – realizing how *easy* it is to
unfold awareness. In time that realization grows into an appreciation that
much of the work dedicated to revealing meaning involves clearing away
the clutter of life – not just of your life, but of all our lives. We all are
obliged to confront, at some point, the clutter and detritus left by others
who have passed through our lives, all leaving their own meanings in
their wake. Not all of us take up that challenge. Perhaps those of us who
shirk the responsibility of clearing up just don't suffer enough. Foolishly,
we fail to recognize the litter status of other people's meanings – our
parents, teachers and other assorted influences. Instead we pick up their
litter, stuffing it like some precious find deep within us, until the treas-

ure of this fool's gold begins to ache as our inner sense recognizes the need to discharge it and get on with the living *our* lives rather than someone else's. The American poet E. E. Cummings (1998) made the pointed observation over 40 years ago that the challenge:

> To be nobody-but-yourself – in a world, which is doing its best, night and day, to make you everybody else – means to fight the hardest battle which any human being can fight; and never stop fighting.

When you began to get a hold on the words that expressed all your sadness, fear and failures, the need to *unfold* awareness began to take precedence. At that point, the whole point of finding *your* point in life made itself manifest. Then and only then, perhaps, you sensed that if you didn't know something that urgently needed knowing, you needed to construct the necessary discourse to help to bring it into awareness – although ultimately the discourse would be not so much with me as with yourself.

Only words

For a long time, words had a terrible power over me, even terrorized me. I was not only afraid of being raped, but afraid to speak the word. Just doing so could induce the fear reaction of the act itself. Names of dead loved ones were unspeakable for the sadness they invoked. It was as if the words themselves were the hurtful things and bore the same threat as the actions or feelings they represented. Constantly being told I would have to speak the words just made me dry up more, feel more fearful, less sure that I would ever be able to comply and more intimidated by the 'presence' of the words. The list of banned words grew as therapy with my counsellor continued and past nightmares reintroduced themselves to my conscious mind. His 'non-directive' approach was experienced as a threatening silence that I felt expected to fill, yet remained completely incapable of doing so. These experiences of word power and threatening silences were reinforced in subsequent meetings with the psychoanalyst, whose method was to encourage me to talk and say little more than 'mmm' herself. These techniques did nothing to help me find a way of expressing myself.

'Mmm' indeed! There is an important assumption that the patient is 'free' to say whatever she wants or needs to say during the golden hour. Almost forty years ago, Shoben expressed the beginnings of a growing concern about how 'non-directive' it was possible for any therapist to be, given the interactive nature of the conversation, far less the intimate relationship engendered within therapy. 'Given the model … of the patient as a computer gone defective, it is ridiculous to talk of … "freedom" granted to the client (sic)' (Shoben, 1963). In Halmos' view, for therapy to be effective it had to be directive in some important way (Halmos, 1981):

> Even in the so-called Uh Huh method of treatment, the therapist's comment is not entirely witheld; at any rate the obviously inevitable physical presence of the therapist-counsellor (sic) will exert its influence in surreptitious ways ... a spontaneous bursting into facial grimace, a nod, a gesture, grunt or sigh, and so on, are utterly inevitable; and even the counsellor's taste in furniture, in clothes, his choice of pictures on the wall of his consulting room, the outward physical signs of his domestic circumstances, the status and other symbols of his consulting room, his publicly reported statements, and several other signs of his activities, will make the ideal of non-directiveness impossible to achieve.

Clearly the truth is that conversations are 'engineered', only sometimes the rationale for this operation is made more manifest than at other times.

Here you raise the thorny issue of *what* exactly we are *expressing*. Different schools of psychiatric thought have different notions about what is *really* going on, *within* the patient. These theories seem to represent little more than different opinions about the nature of reality. If alien anthropologists are studying us, psychotherapy must prove tiresome for these Venusian infiltrators. For despite the internecine struggles between one school of therapy and another, it all must look and sound much the same to the onlooker: two or more people talking. One doing a lot more asking than replying, but still just folks talking. That seems to be just about the beginning and end of *technique* in therapy. The real differences come when the therapists start to attach meanings to the answers that have been generated. Hence the importance of the 'world view' – how the therapist *construes* reality. Of course, some will have no truck with the idea of *construction* of reality in the first place. Things just *are* real, and the patient simply experiences them. This is pretty much on a par with paper and ink: paper just *is* pure and white, and then along comes some ink and scrawls or spatters all over it. There you go, the story of your life, written by reality on your little blank pad of life. Instead, the patient's story reeks of interaction, both past and present. The story spells out vividly how all of us *engage* with reality in such a way that we become lost in the process of engagement, lost in the whole chaotic order of life and living. All our stories echo Yeats' question in 'Among School Children':

> Oh body swayed to music, Oh brightening glance
> How can we know the dancer from the dance? (Adams, 1989)

Stories like yours suggest a quite different scenario. It is true that we all have a story of life being written *as we speak*. However, we play a significant part in the writing of that story. The words aren't just symbols, like typewriter keys. Words do have a powerful presence, for they mean, as Tweedledum and Tweedledee said, pretty much whatever we wish them to mean. Rape may be the name of a dazzling and beautiful rash of colour in the spring countryside (oilseed rape), but it usually has a more malevolent meaning. Much of our language is much less precise, and has a terrific range of *meaning:* happy, successful, want, need, up, flat, addicted, dying, sorted. The meanings of these words can be deduced from the context of the story in which they appear. Sometimes, however, we need to inquire further into what, exactly, the person meant when she said she was happy, or flat, or dying.

The therapist needs to be curious, but in a special way. In particular, there is a need to avoid asking questions to which I suspect I already know the answer. These are not real questions. They are not part of any spirit of genuine inquiry, but are (potentially) just another attempt to manoeuvre the patient. In De Shazer's view, the complex business of asking 'good' questions is what makes therapy, *therapy* (De Shazer, 1994):

> Otherwise doing therapy might become confused with having just any old garden variety conversation.

Wavelengths

The first and most important task for patient and therapist is to find a common language. Most of us have little experience of talking about our thoughts and feelings, and therefore haven't constructed an emotional language. We struggle and are frustrated by our attempts to communicate. I first described this problem to the counsellor, explaining that it seemed as if when I said 'a', he heard 'b'. I received a letter from him giving his view of the problem, which crystallizes what appeared to be happening between us and between myself and subsequent therapists:

> Every client speaks their own language ... As therapists we must learn our clients' language. With some clients this is quite easy, it is similar to our own, with others it is difficult and there is no-one who can translate for us. For me you speak a different language. Never-the-less I feel that I am getting there. I am beginning to speak pidgin-Bobbie.

Sadly we never did find a common language in which we were both fluent. I believe that is what caused him to abandon me. He was simply frustrated by persistent misunderstandings and failure to communicate. I was hard work for no result.

With the analyst, too, there were great gulfs in terms of language as it was spoken and how it appeared to be received by the listener. I soon realized that what I was trying to express was simply not being conveyed by my choice of words. I wanted to shout and scream with frustration, because invariably I perceived the fault to be mine. But on reflection this was not always the case.

You show how there exists a world of difference between listening and hearing. Listening involves just picking up the words and phrases of the story, getting the gist of it, putting ourselves into that story, even. But hearing involves going beyond our simple identification with the other person's story. Hearing involves pushing through to that empathic place where we might gain some appreciation of what it all might mean for the person, even when that meaning seems entirely foreign to us – literally beyond our ken.

Once I recall wanting to fall about laughing at what was clearly, on reflection, an inappropriate response from the psychoanalyst. There had been a gap of several weeks during which I had not seen her. I suppose I was conscious at the start of the session that there would be a little renewing of the relationship necessary, some catching up to be done. In an attempt I think at a jaunty, conversational opener, I breezily asked her: 'Did you miss me, Doc?' She remained silent. I plunged on with 'Like a hole in the head, eh?' There was no recognition of my high spirits and wish to re-establish the relationship on a lighter note. 'Do you feel like a hole in the head?', she asked. I just wanted to burst out laughing. It seemed a totally ridiculous thing to 'reflect back'. What I needed at that point was some chatty dialogue by way of reintroduction to the therapeutic process. Again there seemed to be a breakdown in our communication, but at least on that occasion I experienced the episode as hilarious rather than troubling.

That little scenario leads us to ask what exactly the therapist might be pursuing? What are his assumptions about what needs to be done in therapy? To assume that all psychotherapy abides by the same rules, or that all who aim to help people deal with their troublesome weights have the same ends in mind, is simplistic. The aims of the analyst, the counsellor and the therapist were all quite different, one from the other. In part, this reflected the world views of the professionals themselves and the differing persuasions of their respective schools. It might also reflect something of the people behind the different therapeutic masks. Maybe, different therapeutic approaches attract certain kinds of people. Maybe the 'therapy' only becomes a vehicle for the therapist expressing her or himself.

The history of psychotherapy stretches back to ancient history, through philosopher-priests to the medicine man and magician. That ancient and cross-cultural history may suggest some of the effectiveness of psychotherapy – *why* and *how* it works – which still has much in common with the ideas of the philosophers of religion and the interpersonal skills of the shaman. Indeed, magical, religious and scientific view-points still influence the development of early twenty-first century psy-chotherapies, and are simply three different ways of looking at the same thing – the *mental distress* that we seek to heal.

In this era of evidence-based health care, there is a growing desire to know what 'works' and why. The desire to understand mental healing in a scientific sense began with Freud over a century ago, and continues today with various attempts to analyse and evaluate the interpersonal processes of helping people in mental distress through the power of con-versation – the *talking cure*.

Traditionally, psychotherapy meant the healing of the spirit (or soul). People had a soul sickness that needed some balm, and that balm might be found through unfolding awareness of the possible meanings of the experience of being human. In time, psychotherapy came to mean *the treatment of mental or nervous disorders*. For the analyst, the goal is a 'systematic and total resolution of unconscious conflicts with structural alteration of defences, and the character organization' (Wolberg, 1995).

It shouldn't come as a shock to you to hear that the therapist usually has an investment in the therapeutic method. This is betrayed by the stark differences in style, if not in temperament, between the differing practi-tioners you encountered. The classic analyst favours long silences and long looks; everything means something, usually something significant, otherwise why did the patient care to mention it? Not surprisingly, the analyst failed to appreciate Bobbie's 'sense of humour': why did she need to be so flippant? What exactly was she avoiding?

The classic counsellor is a different animal – oozing empathy, usually hanging onto every word so that it might be reflected back, seeking to provide the conditions under which you might 'know' better the emo-tional significance of that part of your story. If you had encountered tra-ditional behavioural or cognitive therapists, you might have been surprised by the structure that they might have built around and within the conversation.

These are stereotypes, of course, but they suggest not only how differ-ent models of therapy differ on the surface in their methods, but also what expectations these schools have of their practice disciples. Although it is often assumed that therapists practise this or that approach 'because it works', perhaps different approaches attract different people to the practice. The person who spends most of the working day sitting silently behind the free associating patient, may well be naturally inclined to that specific kind of enforced idleness. The therapist who places great store in the organizational structure of behaviour therapy, or in empathic responding, may similarly be revealing more of himself than of the virtues of the method.

Increasingly there is a lot of talk about therapy being 'collaborative', and that through this process the person might somehow be 'empow-ered'. Yet all therapy remains directed by the therapist, even when it is allegedly non-directive. The therapist asks the questions and the person answers. The therapist doesn't answer questions, as the therapist isn't in therapy. It may look like folk talking, but this is no ordinary conversation.

Alternative communication

I have a relative and several friends who have children with learning difficulties. In most cases this involves an underdeveloped language function, but some of the kids have no speech at all. But no words does not mean no communication, and if there's one important thing I've learned from disabled people, it is to concentrate on the things they can do rather than on the things they can't. Similarly, in therapy the important thing is to communicate, so if the patient can't do that with the spoken word (even if for purely psychosomatic reasons) then I think the object should be to find a way she can communicate.

I recall that both the counsellor and the analyst laid great store by the spoken language that passed between us during the hour of therapy. For my own part, I discovered that often the most useful work was done alone, addressing you in letter form, driven by a need to set down and give form to dreams and memories that came flooding back, usually when I was far from your door.

It seems to me that both therapist and patient need to create their own script for therapy and not become locked in a rigid professional method or style. Why is it necessary to face the terrors 'eyeball to eyeball'? Why can we not use alternative means of communication? What's so special about the words spoken during the hour of therapy?

At one extremely traumatic session with the counsellor I ended up having a panic attack, one of the most acute symptoms of which was a locked jaw – a temporary paralysis that for a time left me literally speechless. The counsellor was trying to communicate with me, asking questions, when I caught sight of his laptop computer nearby and made a grab for it, bashing out a basic response with my stiff, tingling fingers.

We never developed the computer as a communication tool, doubtless because it was not deemed sound practice, yet I have always believed this was a wasted opportunity. The laptop was a way into language when I dried up. I found that for some reason it was possible to write things that cannot be spoken. Communication is what's important, not the method of communication. We move on when communication takes place successfully. I no longer have any self-imposed word bans, but that is something that happened naturally when the pressure was off, when I no longer felt under an obligation to say the difficult words out loud before I could claim to be truly 'cured'.

With hindsight, I realize that, far from creating a permanent mute, using alternative forms of communication will eventually lead to actual speech, gently and at the person's own pace. I know some children who use Makaton. The assumption behind this sign language is that they focus on the sign and are less hung up about the noises they make in speech. Eventually, recognizable words are spoken along with the sign.

I have also found other people's attempts to express their feelings a helpful aid to understanding and expressing my own. Sometimes I draw on great literature, sometimes on pop songs. Bruce Springsteen has been just as helpful to me as William Blake. The first time I was able to really express my feelings of loss was by playing a James Taylor track to two very close friends. Music always spoke to me and helped me make some sense of what happened to me and what I was feeling, but I was already in my mid-twenties before I discovered I could share that with anyone else.

When I started with the counsellor and began to let him in, I took the Bruce Springsteen cassette Tunnel of Love *to one of our sessions. I played it a lot at that time, because a lot of the songs on it spoke about conflicting feelings and dichotomies, mirroring my experience of having seemingly diametrically opposing feelings and attitudes raging within me. My favourite song was* Cautious Man*:*

> On his right hand Billy tattooed the word love
> And on his left hand was the word fear
> And in which hand he held his fate was never clear.

If the therapist could explore things like that, it could be a way into building an understanding and a trusting relationship. Once that happens, quietly and without the patient even realizing it has happened, the real speech will come.

Talking Martian on Planet Earth

I also came to appreciate that the words I used didn't always convey the meaning I intended. I would be surprised, even distressed, by the way my words often seemed to get me into deeper trouble. My tortuous attempts to explain my innermost thoughts and feelings often left me feeling more isolated and strange, because it was obvious I was simply not getting through to the listener. Since therapy ended, some subsequent traumas can be put down to a failure in communication. I realize now the power of words, and when something goes wrong in a relationship I try to check very carefully if words were misconstrued, contributing to a breakdown of understanding and sympathy, and to find other words that will serve me better.

I became very troubled when I realized the problem of conveying 'a' when believing I was stating 'b' was likely to be happening many times without my realizing it. Failures of communication were doubtless hap-

pening, and I was carrying on unaware of them. When someone is very upset by something I have said or done, I will realize something is seriously wrong because they are visibly hurt and angry. I will usually not know what the problem is, but I know there is a problem and I must then sit down with the person involved and try very hard to explain myself more adequately and hear what they hear by my words. But there must be many times when the problem is a niggling one and the person lets it pass. The perceived slight is a minor one not considered worth causing a fuss about.

We can't eradicate communication breakdowns, but I think that as both therapists and patients we can try to be more aware of the potential for such problems. Awareness will help us more successfully to avoid problems arising. As listeners, we must try and understand from what position the speaker speaks. A Scotsman declaring 85°F to be 'unbearably hot' would get a puzzled look from an Aborigine used to the 135°F heat of the Australian desert.

The Gospel according to Malcie

I'm interested in how our present understanding of new experiences and information is absorbed according to our constructions of past experiences and information. I'm also very aware of how people may think they are communicating, but actually the receiver has processed the information in a radically different way from that intended by the sender, which can cause real difficulties when both parties are oblivious to this.

During therapy I was much assisted in my development by the insights of a small boy with whom I had regular contact. He was at an age when he was beginning to master the art of the spoken word but was still experiencing basic communication failures. Through his attempts to master everyday language I learned many lessons, which helped in the development of a therapeutic language.

One day Malcie asked me to read him 'the story of the good Somalian', a request that demonstrated the complex way we make sense of incoming information. How could a three-year-old be expected to have any perception of Samaria or its most famous citizen? But he obviously did absorb current news broadcasts, and had some childlike perception of the starving in Africa. So when the story of The Good Samaritan was read to the child, Malcie processed it according to what he already knew, and heard a story about 'a good Somalian'.

With all my therapeutic helpers I experienced 'the good Somalian' syndrome. I feared many things with a fear that seemed exaggerated and inappropriate. I had to learn to reveal past experiences that terrorized me, and how that affected my understanding and response to present experiences. I had to start by using language in a childlike way – some-

times inappropriately and sometimes just not quite right, but under-
standable to a careful listener.

When we explain difficult concepts to children, we often do so by
saying 'It is like ...' and recounting a situation they do understand
through past experience. When a small child asks 'What is thunder?', we
don't recite complex theories of atmospherics. We will offer a simple
explanation, such as 'When the clouds bump into each other, they start to
cry', and this usually satisfies the child until he is ready to accept more
and more detailed, scientific explanations.

The same is true of therapy. We search for meanings we can under-
stand and, at least in the beginning, these can be very simple. We are like
children in our capacity to understand and explain ourselves. Or
perhaps we are like the primitive societies of Biblical times, who grasped
theological concepts through parables.

The journey as a metaphor – the metaphor as a journey

Early in my therapeutic relationship with you we discovered we could
communicate using metaphors. The most enduring metaphors were those
used to describe the process of therapy and the relationship between the
patient and therapist. These early metaphors also carried the seeds of
later, more complex explanations. They somehow had the ability to
develop as my ability to understand the complexities of the therapeutic
process increased.

The first metaphor I remember using successfully was a mountaineer-
ing one. I likened myself to a novice mountain climber. I likened you to
an experienced guide. And so I wrote:

> A climber has to have complete faith in his partner and his equipment. His
> personal safety depends on that. I am aware that I am taking risks with you,
> going into dangerous territory and hoping we will stay safe.

Your use of this metaphor struck a chord with Michael Mahoney's suggestion that therapists might actually cultivate that kind of a relationship
in therapy. Mahoney suggested that if the patient enjoyed reading crime
stories, the therapist might suggest that their relationship be like that of
Sherlock Holmes and Dr Watson. The client had a problem, which was a
mystery. Holmes and Watson set out to solve mysteries. The therapist and
client would set out together to solve this particular mystery.
Mischievously, Mahoney suggested that the client would be Holmes and
he (the therapist) would be his Dr Watson.

Mahoney also made good use of a coach model, which naturally began
to figure strongly in our 'construction' of therapy as I began to appreciate how important 'trying', 'struggling' and 'achieving' was in your life,
mirrored in the sporting side of your personality. And so I gradually

dropped all pretensions as a 'therapist', and became your 'coach'. As Wittgenstein would doubtless have agreed, this was no mere semantic change but a deep reframing of the meaning of our *proper* relationship.

The metaphor began as a simple view of two people making a dogged attempt to complete a difficult task. Later I realized that in therapy the goals are always changing, and what seemed like 'the summit' one month has been scaled by the next month and found to be just another ridge obscuring the view of the way to a higher peak. The metaphor changed with the goals, until finally I was able to conclude that we had only been wandering together 'in the foothills' until I had gained enough experience from my guide and prepared myself well enough to go on to the main assault, a climb that had to be made alone. By this stage I was almost ready to leave therapy.

The likening of therapist and patient to a sports coach and an athlete was also a useful metaphor for our work together. The coach schooled me in techniques and prepared me for the challenges I might face, but I as an athlete had to run the race.

My other useful metaphor for therapy was of patient and therapist at sea in a boat. When therapy begins there is a ferocious storm raging and the therapist is at the helm, using all his strength just to keep the boat from crashing into the rocks and breaking up. At this stage of the process the patient feels out of control, and is desperately looking for someone to 'save' her. I was frustrated by therapists who asked what 'the problem' was, and seemed to seek my advice about how we could solve it. My repeated heartfelt cry was, 'If I knew what to do myself, I wouldn't be asking you'. A developing insight brought the realization that, at the beginning of therapy, therapists are crashing around as much at sea as the patient. Later the picture changes. The storm abates and the boat sails into calmer waters. The metaphor changes, mirroring the therapeutic process. In the latter stages of therapy the boat is becalmed while the therapist listens intently to the patient, who is in control of the boat. Every so often the therapist gently, almost imperceptibly, guides the tiller.

These images encouraged the healing process because you accepted them so enthusiastically. They represented a language that you understood, and further expressed the therapeutic experience in a way you believed would be helpful to other patients. This knowledge, that I had offered something worthy of being passed on to others, was one of the foundations of my reformed self. It was the beginnings of feeling less freakish and less isolated, of rediscovering there was a place for me in the world.

And here the human loop turns back on itself. What else would someone come to therapy for, if not for a glimpse of some of her own inherent worth, of her own intrinsic value? Maybe what you came looking for was validation as a human being, first and foremost.

It is easy to become distracted by the metaphors and metaphorical process of therapy. At its heart lies story framed in language, with two agents trying to make sense of it, rebuilding it and ultimately re-authoring the whole story (White, 1989). The whole conversation between patient and therapist is about words, and neither party has any means other than words to express, represent or even defend themselves. As Confucius observed:

> For one word, a man is often deemed to be wise: and for one word he is often deemed to be foolish. We ought to be careful what we say.

Although the conversation was between you and me, ultimately you ended up talking to yourself – most powerfully, as you discovered – through your journals and letters. The bridge the patient walks across to reach the therapist involves a search for understanding – looking for someone who appears to 'know', humanly, the nature of her distress. Once she has reached that understanding she retraces her steps, having realized (perhaps) that she can lose her mind but, in so doing, come to her senses.

The layperson assumes that mental illness involves some loss of reason – most outrageously when people appear to lose touch with reality. However, this notion is probably wholly false, despite the fact that many professionals subscribe to a similar concept of true madness and the retreat from 'reality'. It seems more appropriate to observe that some people are more aware than others of reality. Reality just *is* for all of us. We can no more lose touch with reality than we can lose touch with the air that supports us. We can, however, lose our awareness of breathing and of air; hence our panic when we think that we cannot breathe and have 'lost' contact with the air. As you began to find the form of words to express something of your experience, you began to develop your awareness of where you were situated in the great reality. As a result, that awareness released reality to begin to work the change process on and through you. All you ever needed to do was to 'unfold awareness', as you so pithily put it. In so doing, you discovered that the rest would come. No mean feat, but an essential one.

By finding an echo of your own voice in mine, you began to make more sense of your story. It is essentially a case of *more* sense, since I believe that your story always made sense. Perhaps it was just not the kind of sense that would satisfy most people. For the story of mental distress often embodies experiences that are untranslatable, because as soon as the patient begins to talk about it she starts cutting up – dismembering – her reality, or feels obliged to add or subtract something to make herself understood. Little wonder that the business of making yourself understood became such a trial for you. Ideas dismantle the whole of the person's experience. As soon as we try to transpose our vision, sense, intuition of 'total experience' of reality into a story with common concepts, the whole thing starts to fragment. Words can give us so much, but they can rarely give us a whole sense of the reality of our experience. They only point, crudely. They act as signposts to that place in our hearts called reality. The finger pointing at the moon should not be confused with the moon itself. Words do have a great power, but much of that power is illusory.

As Mark Twain (1997) observed, 'It was so cold that if the thermometer had been an inch longer, we would all have frozen to death'. This betrays the magic of words – their inherent 'as-if-ness'. Anthony de Mello retold the story of a Finnish farmer who lived on the border with Russia. When the border was being redrawn, he was asked by a Russian official whether he wanted to be in Russia or Finland. Anxious not to upset them, he said ' it has always been my desire to live in mother Russia, but at my age I wouldn't survive another Russian winter' (De Mello, 1995).

Many of us live our lives as if our words had such strange power to change things. In truth, reality just *is*, and all our attempts to represent it are glorious failures. But still we persevere, trying to make ourselves heard and hoping that in so doing we shall be understood. Ultimately we come to the realization that we can no more change ourselves by changing the words we use than we can change our handwriting by changing pens. The story of our lives is really within us, and any change will come from within; it will be an educational experience, as we *educe* the reality of our circumstances.

As our awareness of that core truth grows, we develop what is often called 'insight'. Regrettably, psychiatric professionals talk too much about insight – Have you become more insightful about yourself and your life? I would have to ask you to answer that question, since I can never know another's insight. Such an abstract 'thing' can only be *educed* by the person herself. So when you drew out from within yourself (educed) that realization called 'unfolded awareness', you became your own expert. As you watch yourself, you grow in awareness, picking up feelings and sensations, giving them names, cataloguing them for future reference. Ultimately, you reach a point when you may believe that you have found a way to explain it all. Then, and perhaps only then, do you have to deal with the real villain of the piece – your self-dissatisfaction, your self-condemnation; all those challenges that dislocated you from awareness of reality in the first place. For you always thought that you were more than just words and labels and categories. Now you risk believing, as Sullivan noted, that 'the self is largely a verbal edifice'.

Maybe you learned that language is alive and growing, and is not permanent. Through that lesson you may have unpicked the riddle of the change process: that, as Confucius observed, 'the one who would be constant in happiness must constantly change'. You discovered that it is not simply the case that nothing lasts – that all truths are provisional – but also that your story is itself in flow. Like the words you use to express it, it is not a static thing that can be 'caught' in words or phrases, far less by the terminology of psychobabble. It is living in every phrase that trips from your tongue or scrawls from your pen. There is no goal to reach; reaching is its own goal.

References

Adams, H. (1989). *The Book of Yeats Poems*. Florida State University Press.
Boldt, L. G. (1997). *Zen Soup*, p. 70. Arkana.
Cummings, E. E. (1998). *AnOther*. W. W. Norton
De Mello, A. (1995). *Awareness*. Fount.
De Shazer, S. (1991). *Putting Differences to Work*. W. W. Norton.
De Shazer, S. (1994). *Words were originally Magic*, p. 96. W. W. Norton.
Gay, P. (1995). *The Freud Reader*, p. 37. Vintage.
Halmos, P. (1981). *The Faith of the Counsellors*, pp. 94–5. Constable.
Illich, I. (1976). *Medical Nemesis: The Expropriation of Health*. Marion Boyars.
Peplau, H. E. (1969). Psychotherapeutic strategies. *Perspect. Psychiatric Care*, **6,** 264–70.
Shoben, E. J. (1963). The therapeutic object: men or machines? *J. Cons. Psychology*, **10,** 3.
Sullivan, H. S. (1953). *The Interpersonal Theory of Psychiatry*. W. W. Norton.
Todorov, T. (1984). *Mikhail Bakhtin: The Ideological Principle* (translated by W. Godzich), p. 30. The University of Minnesota Press.
Twain, M. (1997) *Speeches*. Oxford University Press.
White, M. (1989). *Selected Papers*. Dulwich Centre Publications.
Whorf, B. L. (1956). *Language, Thought and Reality*. John Wiley and Sons.
Wittgenstein, L. (1965). *The Blue and Brown Books: Preliminary Studies for the 'Philosophical Investigations'*, p. 28. Harper.
Wolberg, L. R. (1995). *The Technique of Psychotherapy*, p. 5. Jason Armstrong.

5

Mutuality

Life is like setting sail in a boat that we all know is going to sink someday.

Suzuki Roshi

The unreasonable relationship

We may deny it, we may even construct all sorts of metaphors about professional *distance* and the need for *boundaries*, but life is an event that we are all in together. However much I might like to think that the patient's distress is alien to my experience, this is just another play on words, for life is an ocean of experience and we all get wet sooner or later. No one said it more elegantly than Harry Stack Sullivan when he remarked that 'we are all more simply human than otherwise' (Sullivan, 1953). It is worth noting that Sullivan saw no difference, in human terms, between the experience of people who were described as 'psychotic' and his own experience. Crazy they might well be, to the layperson and even to many professionals, but to Sullivan this was just another way of 'being human', perhaps under the most awesomely 'inhuman' conditions. It was no accident either, perhaps, that as an analyst in the late 1930s he abandoned the traditional technique of sitting silently behind his patients. Instead, he moved his chair to sit alongside, as if to demonstrate that he too was in the soup along with them. And so began the collegiality of minds that led to what we now, more prosaically, call the 'therapeutic alliance'[1].

---

[1]Although the 'therapeutic' or 'working alliance' had its origins in psychoanalysis, to many analysts this was a shady deal offered by the analyst to gain the patient's compliance (Brenner, 1976).

The tradition of the psychoanalytic method from which Sullivan was trying to escape over 70 years ago possessed, in Malcolm's view (Malcolm, 1982):

> a radical unlikeness to any other human relationship, its purposeful renunciation of the niceties and decencies of ordinary human intercourse, its awesome abnormality, contradictoriness and strain.

A significant part of that psychoanalytic practice involved the physical relationship between analyst and analysand. This stereotype of 'therapy', with the silent, thoughtful and half-hidden analyst skulking behind the patient, has become known to several generations of non-patients through the medium of film; not least the comic realities of New York life portrayed by Woody Allen. We have long since forgotten, if indeed many of us ever knew, that the traditional practice of psychoanalysis, in which the analyst situated himself *behind* the patient, was borne primarily of Freud's 'dislike of being stared at all day' (Malcolm, 1982). The therapeutic method originally developed by Freud had obvious associations with confession, including the interpersonal distance between the patient and her 'father confessor'. Significantly, Sullivan stepped outside of that cloistered role and, in getting closer to the patient (humanly as well as physically), announced the beginnings of therapy through the means of 'interpersonal relationships'. The highly unpredictable nature of such 'interpersonal relations' is the substance of this chapter.

The unpredictability of all our lives is perhaps the thing we deny most. Some part of us never wants to grow up. Some part of us tries to remain like that kid from our memory who wants to stay out late, playing long after the sun has dropped below the horizon. Little wonder that many of us have slipped so easily into that culture of sun-worshippers, who flit off to sandy beaches and cheap plonk as soon as the seasons turn their cold backs to our faces. Having grown up and lived all my life in a land of four very clearly defined seasons, the notion of exchanging them for sunshine on tap seems not only profligate, but also lies close to surrendering my own spirit. I was born for the unpredictability of British weather, so why should I resist its unpredictability?

Yet people often resist themselves in the same way. Maybe all that searching for sun, sangria and sex is just part of that self-denial. Maybe the search for the certainties of summer is a mirror image of our attempts to distance ourselves from human uncertainty. Dissatisfaction breeding disaffection. In everyday practice, we deny our human chaos through our vain attempts to control our lives. They are vain in both senses of the word, since these struggles connote our failure to recognize futility when we should know it in our very bones. This also has something to do, perhaps, with our foolish belief that *we* can achieve anything worthwhile. Plutarch recognized this when he was alleged to have said:

> So we in all casualties of life should say, 'I knew my riches were uncertain,
> that my friend was but a man'. Such considerations would soon pacify us,
> because all our troubles proceed from their being unexpected.

He had, of course, doubtless thought long and hard about the impermanence of life, and had long since faced up to the fact that 'life itself
decays, and all things are daily changing'. Arguably, this is the only true
fact of life. Such constant change is something we would rather not
acknowledge. We talk much about wanting to 'go back' to some glory
days or golden time when we were happy, contented and free of anxiety,
or before we ever learned the meaning of the experience of *angst*. But
such going back is not possible. Indeed, as Plutarch observed, 'it is unreasonable to expect an exemption from the common fate'. But expect it we
invariably do. When patients first come to therapy, most expect that
through some process of expiation they will be relieved of the burden of
their distress, and will be exempt from any future distress. Indeed, the
commonest answer to the question, 'what do you hope to gain from
therapy?' is 'to go back to the way I was before!' Perhaps patients adopt
this view because of the level of their distress, or perhaps it is simply that
they are more honest than most of us, who also would dearly love to be
able to 'confess' ourselves into some state of certain bliss.

Coming together

Alan Watts (1993) retold a lovely Persian tale about a sage who died and
went to heaven. When he knocked on heaven's door:

> From within the voice of God asked, 'Who is there?', and the sage
> answered, 'It is I'. 'In this House,' replied the voice, 'there is no room for
> thee and me'. So the sage went away, and spent many years pondering over
> this answer in deep meditation. Returning a second time, the voice asked
> the same question, and again the sage answered, 'It is I'. The door remained
> closed. After some years he returned for the third time, and at his knocking
> the voice once more demanded, 'Who is there?' And the sage cried, 'It is
> thyself!'. The door was opened.

When the patient meets the therapist, what *exactly* is agreed? Is it reasonable to expect that one should *heal* the other? But on the other hand,
is it reasonable to expect that the therapist should simply remind the
patient of her unreasonableness in expecting 'an exemption from the
common fate'? It seems obvious that the therapist should aim, at least, to
prove (eventually) that he could be *helpful*. In being helpful, he may help
himself. The irony that Freud found it difficult to face (physically) his
patients, who found it difficult to face (metaphorically) themselves,
should not be lost on us. The distance between patient and therapist is an

illusory space. We are like one, as were the sage and God (though we know not which we might be). The relationship becomes, almost immediately, like a dance, as patient and therapist *conjoin*. Having come together in some form of human unity, healing of psychic pain is high on the agenda. Yet healing is either something that (just) happens or, more likely, is something that goes on within the person being healed. Therapists, whatever they care to believe, don't heal or even 'fix' or 'sort' anything, but merely provide the conditions that appear necessary for these abstract and often ephemeral processes to take place[2]. And, of course, one function of the relationship is to facilitate that self-healing, although what exactly might be the 'self' that is healed, and who or what might play a part in healing it, remains one of the eternal therapeutic riddles.

What exactly do we mean when we talk of therapists 'helping' the self-healing process along? Alan Watts reminded us of the dangers of being too helpful (Watts, 1991):

> Kindly let me help you or you'll drown' said the monkey, putting the fish safely up a tree. The moment you take this attitude of 'you are sick', people learn to eat pity, and thrive on it, and play sick as a profitable role for getting attention, sympathy, care and to indulge in the masochism of gaining a sense of identity through being in peril, in misfortune.

The monkey illustrates the problem of being 'too caring', and Watts appears to be warning us to watch out for such 'monkeys', who might encourage us to believe that the emotional rescue they offer will not, ultimately, be the spiritual death of us.

You reflected in your journal on something very close to this paradox.

There is a charity called Six Circle, which has as its motto, 'By meeting the needs of others, we meet our own'. The charity brings together young offenders, disabled people and disadvantaged families with others who have no obvious needs and social or emotional disadvantages. They join together for social activities and outings, knowing that everyone gets something from the experience, finds it personally as well as communally beneficial.

There is an honesty there about need and interdependence that I didn't find in my therapeutic encounters. Yet it seems obvious to me that the therapist does seek to meet his or her own needs in the therapeutic encounter. That isn't necessarily a negative comment. For any relationship to continue and develop, each of the partners in the relationship has

---

[2]Almost twenty years ago a colleague introduced me to a Greek scholar at the University of St Andrew's, who helped me coin a simple Greek neologism for 'the necessary conditions for the promotion of growth and development' – *trephotaxis*. Although uncertain of many things, I am fairly certain that when therapists can be *trephotarcs,* their patients begin to feel the healing happen within them.

to be finding something positive for themselves in that relationship. The trick is to be aware of what we need for ourselves and what others need from us, matching the needs in a successful relationship.

I am well aware that my relationship with you was successful not only because you were able to help me to acquire some basic coping skills and encourage personal development, but also because I presented as an interesting case through whom you could extend your professional expertise. You were getting something from our therapeutic meetings too. I don't think either of us has a problem acknowledging that. I don't feel manipulated now, nor did I then. Nor do I feel there was an imbalance of dependency.

Recognizing that now, though, doesn't mean that I think it either helpful or desirable for the patient to be focused on the needs of the therapist during therapy. The person in therapy has enough to cope with without that heavy burden. The very reason people go into therapy at all is because they can't cope with their own problems. They don't need to go looking for any more.

But any attempt to assess what is appropriate and inappropriate therapy has to consider motive and gain for the therapist. Why do therapists do what they do? Is there a danger that a drive to meet their own needs will override the drive to meet the patients' needs? I believe that, in some cases, the answer to the latter question is undoubtedly yes.

When I was seeing the counsellor, I remember asking how long he thought our therapeutic relationship would last. There was a practical reason for the question – I was finding it increasingly difficult to meet the costs as therapy went on and my finances dwindled. Emotionally I became hooked into the relationship and felt I needed him and couldn't end the relationship, yet practically I looked to a time when I could stand alone and end the regular financial commitment. He told me some clients were in therapy for a couple of years; one had spent four years in therapy and another seven. I knew I couldn't cope financially with such a protracted relationship.

Of course therapists – even counsellors – have to eat and pay the mortgage, but I think that I get your drift. Ideally, human helping should be given freely – a gift. Even those who value the importance of being 'unconditional' invariably make conditions. Paying for help is not simply a part of the market culture that now floods every area of our lives, but is part of the legacy of psychoanalysis. Freud was the first to argue that the patient should pay even for missed appointments. He was locating the responsibility for the 'work' of therapy squarely in the patient's territory. The growth of your dependence on the counsellor shows just how similar to ordinary relationships therapy can be. Which is why, perhaps, therapists and counsellors develop techniques and structures to contain some of that; to protect themselves from their own ordinariness.

The graceful relationship

Therapy is, of course, no ordinary relationship. Indeed, what strains the seams of the normal relationship, such as friendship or marriage, to bursting point may even be a necessary part of the relating that is called therapy. Relationships don't work. People within relationships make them work, or maybe it is just the people who 'work' or 'don't work'. Relationships that we classify as successful may simply reflect the actions of people who make the whole business of relating look easy. Whether or not therapists tell their clientele that this is likely, or even desirable, is another matter. Perhaps therapists are loath to admit the extent to which therapy might mirror life, or *vice versa*. As Thomas Moore argued so powerfully (Moore, 1994):

> Relationship is not a project, it is a grace. The difference between these two is infinite, and since our culture prefers to make everything a project, to be accomplished with effort and understanding, to be judged pure failure when it doesn't arrive at the expected conclusion, it is not easy to treat intimacy as grace.

I do not wish to appear falsely naïve when I say that I never really *knew* what was happening within our relationship. It was an experience that was alive, organically growing between us, yet belonging to neither of us alone. I have written elsewhere of my appreciation of how my life has been graced by people entering my world in the guise of patients. It was no different with you, despite the fact that you are now far away in time, and perhaps also quite distant in terms of our original 'grace notes'[3]. These kind of reflections will be read by some as 'mushy' if not anachronistic yearnings for a form of therapy that might be seen to have died with the end of the '60s project', triggered by the emergence of humanistic therapy at the end of the 1950s. Such criticisms may, however, only add further evidence to Moore's concern that life has become a 'total project' and what we are 'dealing with' or 'addressing' or trying to 'resolve' has become lost from our vision. We can *see* what needs to be done, but we have lost the vision that might see beyond our immediate world of difficulties and problems.

Perhaps therapists simply let the relationship 'develop' as an easy option. This suggests its organic nature; both are required to deal with the tensions, as and when they arise. You experienced just such a tension when you were obliged to confront the possibility that your counselling relationship wasn't working.

There was a reluctance to decide counselling wasn't working, having spent a small fortune in fees. I felt I wasn't making progress, but didn't

---

[3]It is notable that, unsolicited, you included MacLaverty's (1998) *Grace Notes* in your section in Chapter 9.

want to waste my 'investment' when for all I knew improvement was just around the corner. But, on the other hand, I didn't want to continue throwing good money after bad. Which was it to be?

There seemed to be only one person who could advise me – the counsellor! However, with hindsight I realize he was hardly an impartial judge. He too had a lot to lose. Financially, he would lose my regular income. Indeed, one of my friends suggested that I was making payments on his family holiday to the USA. He also had a lot to lose professionally. He saw himself as a skilled counsellor who had not, thus far, had to give up on a case. He had to admit to himself that, in taking me on as a client, he might have bitten off more than he could chew.

When I did put my quandary to him, he discussed what he saw as 'progress' with me and took the view that I should continue, but also said that the decision was always mine. In reality, I wondered, was I really able to make such a decision? What was truly 'in my best interests'? Was I right to concede, as I do now from this distance, that, far from being an equal relationship, I gave far more weight to his opinion and expertise than might have been healthy? Could the decision to continue really be described as an informed one, made by me alone? Did he manipulate the trust I had placed in him? He said that the choice was mine, but he must have known that he had the power to persuade me to continue.

In my view, what took place three or four months after this momentous decision to continue was nothing short of abuse. Having decided to 'go for it', committing myself heart and soul to the therapy, the counsellor then took the decision independently to bail out. This was a decision that was absolutely not up for discussion between the two allegedly 'equal' partners in the therapeutic relationship. I certainly did not believe at the time that it was best for me, and threw a tantrum that any two-year-old would have been proud of. The counsellor still left, after having collected his fee.

I can sympathize with your frustration, but also feel for the hapless counsellor. I wonder, if he had been 'highly qualified' and 'full time', would it have been any different? Traditionally, we have excused psychoanalysts all manner of things. Charles Brenner once addressed the issue of what to do if the analyst dozed off during the session and the patient refused to pay. In his view, the analyst should neither apologize nor protest, but should continue with the analysis, inquiring into the processes (of the patient) that might 'lie behind' his refusal to pay, and his 'anger towards the analyst'. Since we appear to have decided, as a society, that analysis is largely bunkum, we may laugh at this attempt at psychoanalytic reassurance. However, the story does contain an important kernel of reality. The time is always the patient's time, even when therapists steal it by trying to examine or explore only that which they wish to explore.

The differences between your accounts of the counsellor and the analyst suggest two different views of, obviously, two very different people. Perhaps you excused the analyst all manner of things – such as her getting lost in 'her frantic, silent, note-taking' – because she was highly qualified, though in what exactly you didn't know. As I mentioned above, people came to expect this from classical psychotherapy; they knew no better and did not protest. People came to expect the analytic relationship to be largely lacking in most of the ordinary niceties of human intercourse. However, given the avowedly human dimension of the counselling project, perhaps you had higher expectations of the counsellor, despite his lowly status in the psychiatric power game. Yet another paradox.

Terms of engagement

These reflections on the nature of the relationship that developed between us, and indeed between you and your other therapists, prompted a consideration of what might be called the 'terms of engagement'. And so, you write:

Finding a form of address that both the patient and therapist are comfortable with must be one of the first tasks of the therapeutic encounter. Initially I always referred to the counsellor as Mr, though he always used my first name and encouraged me to do likewise. Similarly, I always referred to the analyst as Doctor. I think that my preference for a formal mode of address was my natural resistance to what I would call the 'immediate friends' syndrome. It takes time to build a relationship based on genuine respect and approval. I realize that many therapists will operate by trying to show that they are sympathetic and care deeply for their patients. However, to the ordinary person like me, it can come across as a false pose, a professional technique, and pretty valueless at that.

I went through something of the same with you. At the start of our association I preferred to use the formal address 'Dr Barker', because I got a lot of security from the professional title. The title assured me that I was dealing with someone who was qualified and would have methods to solve my problems, not simply someone offering a listening ear, who might be as lost as I was when it came to facing my problems. The formal title also helped my mind to distance the professional therapist from the counsellor with whom I had previously had such a bad experience.

As I started to become more relaxed and allowed myself to get to know you better, I preferred to use 'coach', which was a less formal title but still denoted a job, and suggested a clearly defined relationship. Over time, it just happened that I was able to accept you (the therapist) as yourself, and it felt right to use your Christian name. By then we had begun to have a more relaxed, friendly association, and I had

already begun the process of preparing to leave the therapeutic relation-
ship.

When we began writing this chapter, I asked you why, in your letters and
journal notes, you had always referred to the analyst as 'Doc'. Perhaps
because of the association with Bugs Bunny, I had assumed that this was
a term of endearment, or at least a sign that the relationship had its lighter
side. This was far from the truth, as you saw it:

When you asked me about my use of the term 'Doc', I quite reeled when
you described it as 'almost affectionate'. I had no sense of who the
analyst was. A friend of mine who was a doctor's wife told me that the
analyst was married to someone who was pretty well-known, and that she
had a daughter. These brief details helped me to paint some kind of a
human picture of her. Had I not had that input I feel that the 'relation-
ship' would have been even more tortuous than it was, for the 'Doc' gave
absolutely nothing away. I think I was always trying to get her to hang
loose, just to speak to me, make me feel more at ease and less of a psy-
chiatric case. However, all her psychiatric poses militated against this. I
think my use of the term 'Doc' was part of my trying to humanize her and
our relationship. Without even realizing it at the time, I was trying to put
us in the position of being, as you would say, 'just two people making
themselves up as they talked'. Also, I think it was something to do with
preparing to share very intimate, hurtful and frightening things with
someone who, in truth, was a total stranger. Maybe it was my attempt to
make her more like some kind of confidante, which was what I was being
asked to do: confide. *But it's difficult to be so open, vulnerable and*
sharing with a blank face.

Although there exists a huge and largely contradictory literature about
the *role* of the therapist, over the years my confusion about what exactly
I needed to be doing has been mostly resolved. In my therapeutic youth,
like many others, I strove to *know* something about people in general that
I might apply to people in particular – like you. In time, I grew to appreciate that there was no-one like you, or any other 'patient' for that matter.
I came to value the privilege of studying (if you like) uniqueness – or
rather, participating in the exchange of our mutual uniqueness.

The trouble with expert knowledge is that it assumes to *know* (obviously) what is good, normal and worthy of being valued. We affirm that
anxiety is bad and relaxation is good. End of story! Under these therapeutic rules, the therapist is responsible for working out what is 'wrong'
with the patient and, having made this formulation, for working out how
to treat the symptoms of the problem, or even the source of the problem
itself. Such problem-based approaches to people and the whole complex
business of living require, of course, a corresponding assumption about
human pathology. Therapists like me who view 'anxiety' and 'relaxation'

more simply – as ways of being at the moment – also recognize that such ways of being might have a function; one that we should be careful about removing, at least too quickly[4].

I came to the conclusion about fifteen years ago that such an approach to 'therapy' didn't make sense. Now I appreciate better that 'therapy' is simply a linguistic construction. All those years ago, I was being disturbed by something that was going on within my relationships with patients that I did not understand but could undeniably 'feel'. I had spent, at that time, over five years working closely with women who were diagnosed as depressed or psychotic or both. Invariably their family members looked to me for reassurance or validation of the 'madness' they had to live with. The longer I spent with these women the more I grew to appreciate the meaningfulness of their troubled existence, and the more difficulty I encountered in relating to the appeals of the spouses (especially) who wanted their mad partners 'treated'. I took this to mean, perhaps wrongly, that they wanted their wives and partners 'silenced'. Or, at least, they wanted the mad voice that troubled them from time to time to be silenced.

Therapy is just two people talking. If one attempts to silence the other, the conversation ends, prematurely and possibly acerbically. I experienced some kind of an attenuated epiphany over those years in therapy with those women. I have often thought that I was the greater beneficiary of those encounters. I learned there that it is not possible to be 'objective' about a person's life or their experience of life. I learned that it is my privilege to be a partial witness to that experience, and it is folly to assume that I might have privileged access to what that experience, far less that whole life, might mean in terms of its human value. I learned there the importance of approaching the story that unfolds in therapy with respect and also with curiosity. I know virtually nothing of any note about the person. It is my privileged task to take some instruction from the patient about the nature, function and meaning of her or his life. Although I discount the idea that I might be any kind of an expert on the patient's life, I recognize my role as a facilitator of a conversation that might lead to new possibilities in that life. In that sense, my role is an important if not a powerful one. I try to give that power the respect it deserves.

Curious change

And so I became more curious – or I appeared to rediscover the (almost idle) curiosity that first brought me into the field (Barker, 1999). The fol-

[4]In challenging the notion that such phenomena were symptoms of 'mental illness', Szasz affirmed that instead they were merely 'problems of living', a term first coined by Harry Stack Sullivan. Whether the patient ostensibly has a 'choice' is an irrelevance, since choice – with its very special meaning – distracts us from the issue raised by Szasz and Sullivan. These ways of being are meaningful expressions of how the person is 'working'. They are, in effect, strategies for living.

lowing extract from your journal was typical of your response to my 'curiosity' about what was happening within your world of experience, a curiosity that extended beyond the boundary of the consulting room.

Friday, July 17 4.15 pm

Dear Coach,

Right now I'm on the train on my way to London for the bike run. I am aware of the question in your letter, which was something along the lines of 'was I changing or was I just noticing change more?' I would say a bit of both. Though I was struck dumb yesterday afternoon when you asked how I'd got on with the homework. It wasn't because I hadn't been think-ing about it. I'd actually done quite a bit of work, but I couldn't see how I could explain change and noticing change without giving a long expla-nation spanning a number of years of experience.

You have said you are not really interested in what happened in the past, only what's happening now and where I want to get to in the future. That's fine. In fact, in months gone by, knowing that has given me more confidence as I don't feel with you that the bad things are lurking there waiting to jump out and break me when you decide it's time to push me into progress. I think progress has come from the feeling it will not be forced.

Just the same, each time I thought about your 'riddle' I would think about people I have known and how my feelings and attitudes towards them have changed over a period of time. To offer you an answer, it seemed that I would have to give a sort of emotional history. A lot of it at the moment seems to come from what I see as my particularly bad expe-rience of 'therapy'. Maybe it's wrong, or just plain tedious from your point of view, but I think I need to write down all of that, and it did have an adverse effect on one particular relationship, before I can purge myself of C (the counsellor) and put all that behind me.

Therapists don't do much more than ask questions, although not all ques-tions are what I would call 'curious questions' – where the therapist really doesn't know the answer and is not (subtly) leading the patient. Some of the questions that appeared to stick in your memory were the 'sticky ones', perhaps the most curious ones of all. You say elsewhere that I showed (and perhaps also confessed) little interest in your past, the whole 'history' of your difficulties. That is true, and also serves to dis-tinguish the kind of therapy that took place between us from, at least, some other forms of therapy. The focus of our relationship was on 'con-structing reality' as we spoke. In one very specific sense, neither you nor I had any history; only a story *about* our history, which we edited accord-ing to context. I was more interested in helping you to write on the present (blank) page of your life storybook. My occasional follow-up letters, which carried my reflections on our co-creation of therapeutic reality, were aimed at continuing that conjoint 'reality making' across the ether. If you like, I was more interested in the possibilities for what you might become (future) than I was interested in the confirmation of what you might have been (history). When you were distressed, or talking about distress, it was important to ask, 'what is that (distress) like or about?' or 'what does it do to you?' Most times, however, we moved on swiftly to talk about what it might be like to be different – How would you know that things were different? What experience had you already had of being different? And so we came to such curious questions as, 'how do you know you are changing, rather than just noticing change more?'

Wednesday, October 28 1.20 pm

Dear Coach,

I got your letter this morning, which has bucked me up. Thanks. It wasn't the content that did it, because I am all at sea with that, it was just nice to get a letter. I had been feeling really exasperated with you – well, no, that's not right. It comes out that I am really exasperated with you, but I think really it's more about me being exasperated with me.

I have pointedly avoided doing my book work because I was very unsettled about how things were going. I was very frustrated that I wasn't progressing – that is, I was still struggling with thoughts I have been thinking for years and I felt I should have them sussed by now.

Shoulds and should nots is one of the no-nos. Right? I read that when I skimmed your self-help guide.

I think partly I have been avoiding the book work to avoid creating further frustration and anxiety with myself faced with what seems to me to be a demonstrable lack of progress. But even this seems predictable behaviour, as I came across a bit in your book which says something like, patients getting annoyed when they seem to take a backward step is in fact a sign of progress.

Another part of the difficulty that made me retreat is that there was a big problem I have been thinking a lot about, especially since a visit to my cousin last week and things she said to me, but I just couldn't bring myself to write it down on paper and have it on record. I would like to be able to tell you about it, but it is too dangerous a thing to be on permanent record.

I have been being a bit of a prat, trying to put a distance between myself and all this, kid on for a couple of weeks that there's no real hassle, nothing I can't handle. Well, at the end of the day I suppose that is true, but that is not realized or achieved by ignoring what I'm thinking or feeling.

The thing that gets me is here I am trying to be positive and develop helpful attitudes and often, in the midst of my big thinks, all I am really certain of is how uncertain I am about anything. I think I've got something or someone sussed and adopt a helpful attitude, and then for no apparent reason that changes.

But maybe this is all there is. Maybe that's what you're trying to help me to do – realize there are no absolute responses, ways of behaving faced with certain situations and learning to just go with the flow and adopt what seems the right response at the time, even if that's different from the last time. And nothing is completely the same anyway, is it? When I was so upset last time I saw you, I had this feeling I wanted to crawl under the table and it would be safe. Part of me wanted to tell you all about what that felt like, but another part of me was fighting against that because a couple of years ago I had that same feeling and told somebody else, so I was feeling that too and trying to keep him out of the cupboard and separate from you, but when I'm on automatic pilot it gets mixed up and I can't separate people. I think you were getting a response from me that rightly was for somebody else. Well, anyway, I know what I mean, but it must be awful hard for you to follow.

This morning too I was so swamped because when I got your letter first it bucked me up and made me want to do some work for you. I decided I was going to read your book from cover to cover and glean the right way forward! Also I had to read ALL the papers on the child abuse stuff, as well as the past week of papers, which I have only had time to glance at. This is meant to be my day off, yet I got myself in a panic because I wasn't reading quickly enough or absorbing enough of what I was reading. After TWO HOURS of reading a paper over and over, I realized this wasn't helping me at all. I have now decided NOT to keep papers piling up 'til I've read them properly. The plan is that at the start of each day I will read what I reasonably can before getting on with the day. If I have moments during the day when I can pick up articles that specifically interest me, fine. But I won't HAVE TO read all the papers. Every day will be a new day, starting fresh. Papers will be thrown out at the end of each day, so there's not a load of stuff carried over to daunt me at the start of each new day. Mind, this has not to be an excuse to do nothing and withdraw totally, as I did with the book work these last two weeks, but it seems to make sense to start and say 'I've accomplished this and this today', which is more helpful than 'I didn't manage to do this, this, this and this today'. When I think about it this is no great revelation, though it feels like it to me. It's really what you say in your book, isn't it? But I learn things better if I experience them rather than just read about something abstract. I think that's why Kopp meant nothing to me when I was first introduced to him, and now he's a right-on bloke.

I have just read your letter again. I am so slow. I have only just twigged that 'guilt is just a superficial glitter' is a wordplay on gilt. Mind you, I still can't figure it out. I can't think of anything I said in the letter to you that has brought this on, so maybe you had better bring it next time so I can match up the two and maybe get 'perfect sense'. I don't think!!

If I was helping to prepare you for anything, it was to become your personal philosopher. Gradually you began to ask yourself the kind of questions I had been asking you. You gradually took over the whole process of therapy, and I gradually became redundant. I always knew you would, since almost from the first moment you began to talk I knew that within 'you' there was a 'you' (1) who was able to watch, take note, and generally make judgements about 'you' (2). There were at least two 'yous' operating: one of them (the watcher) appeared to work perfectly, and the other (the watched) was judged to be weak and problematic, along with a whole range of other negatives. In that sense you (1 and 2) were pretty much like me and everybody else. The difference was that you (1) gradually closed the connection with you (2) and, in so doing, Bobbie became one (almost). When you began to notice how you lost your awareness of yourself (became less self-aware) and got lost in the business of living – whether cycling, brushing your teeth or listening to music – you began to heal the rift within yourself: a rift which is part of the downside of thinking and feeling. If my approach had any core philosophy, it involved the recognition that someone who knew they had a problem – even a thousand problems – already had the answer tucked up within their 'self'. That answer lay within 'you (1)' who had 'noticed' the problem in the first place.

My letters were important, and not simply as messages of support or affirmation – which were important in their own right. They were important as a means of maintaining the philosophical dialogue that had begun days earlier in the consulting room. Your journal entry above shows how your philosophical work was a bit of a roller coaster. You struggled and then you rested, and then began to give in to some of the experiences, and then struggled some more. If I had been there – fly on the wall-style – I might have asked, 'what is it like?', or 'how do you keep coming back for more?', or 'are you swimming with the current or against it?', or 'how far have you travelled? If you had said, as you sometimes did, 'no distance at all!', I might have asked, 'so how do you keep going? Where do you get the courage/motivation/strength/guts (or whatever) to keep going?'.

Do you remember me asking some of those damn fool silly questions? And of course, sometimes I simply asked one question too many. I have a tendency to work too hard at being the therapist.

Relationship through the mirror

One day you wrote a long letter about one of your friends, who was intending to train as a counsellor. It sounded as if you kept your counsel, but the story that unfolded stirred up some difficult feelings for you.

My friend, who I feel I have been losing over recent months, asked me to play badminton today. She mentioned that her counselling course that she is going on next month is going to be ratified by the university. Obviously I was meant to be impressed.

Your friend's ambition to become a counsellor drew her close, in your mind, to your bad experience of counselling. Perhaps that reflection prompted your own reflection on the nature and status of your relationship with your old friend.

What I 'notice'[5] about M is that there are bits of her that I don't like. I don't like her counselling work and I also think that I can't admire her (totally) any more.

What I have to work out is if there is still enough left to be friends, or will the bad bits take over. Partly I think that the answer lies in numbers 17 and 18 on the laundry list[6]. I can see that I have a tendency to idolize people, have intense friendships for a period and then feel let down when the feeling wanes and I become more aware of their human failings than their superior status. Maybe I just have to accept that real closeness is a passing state that will not last forever. The trick is (I think) to enjoy it to the full when you have it, but don't try to hang on to it when its gone. Not that it is possible to do that anyway. Once it's gone, it's gone. No amount of willing things back the way they were brings them back. And the laundry list says you can't make somebody love you. My addition to that is that you can't make yourself love somebody else. Blake (Stevenson, 1989) had it right when he said:

> He who binds to himself a joy
> Does the winged life destroy
> He who kisses the joy as it flies
> Lives in Eternity's sunrise.

You had only just 'discovered' Kopp and his laundry list the day before, and in your journal you had written:

---

[5]I noticed that you emphasized that you were 'noticing'. This was a fine illustration of how you had turned simple 'reflection' into a kind of 'meditation *in* life'.

[6]A reference to Sheldon Kopp's *Eschatological Laundry List: A Partial Register of the 927 (or was it 928) Eternal Truths*. I had suggested to Bobbie that she might find this interesting reading, and she appeared to study it religiously, recognizing – as Kopp intended – the irony of employing a laundry list of truths in such an uncertain universe. No. 17 stated: 'There are no great men' and No. 18 advised: 'If you have a hero, look again: you have diminished yourself in some way' (Kopp, 1974).

Dear Fellow Pilgrim[7]

I have discovered Kopp and am struggling not to lionize him. He is hero material, but of course he is right (see 17 and 18 on the Laundry List).

Though I had already discovered the list for myself in your book (Barker, 1992), I thank you for this 'therapeutic gift". I hear what you are saying to me, and I am not afraid. I shall miss you, but I am not afraid. Most of what I need is in myself. If I keep looking I will find it. Thank you for guiding me through the foothills. We are almost at the base of the mountain, and when we reach it I shall say goodbye and not look back. My face will turn up to the summit. Thank you for preparing me for the climb.

In one of our final conversations, I had exercised some 'caution' concerning reading about the self and the whole complex business of living and relating[8]. Earlier that afternoon a patient had asked me quite directly what I thought of something. It was a searching question, one that I felt I could not simply return. Rather than answer in words, I said 'it seems like …' and drew a little picture on the pad. She smiled and said, 'I see … you are quite the little Leonardo'. It is a rare occurrence for a therapist to be ridiculed so gently by a patient. I must have basked in this comment, which was as unusual as it was ordinary. I thought of Leonardo again, perhaps, because of his dislike of books. Arguably one of the greatest minds in the Western world believed that we should not contaminate our thinking with the thoughts of others. Instead, we should go out and study the world directly. You were not quite ready for that and, quite rightly, said so. I was striking the wrong balance, trying to push you rather than allow you to continue pulling me.

I hear what you say about reading, but don't go the whole way with you on that. You fear I will substitute book learning for experience, but I don't think it's the best way to steer completely clear of the former in favour of the latter. As with many other things in life, what's needed is a proper balance. I have wondered why books have started to be important to me again, and meaningful. I conclude it is because what I choose to read gives an echo of my own experience. Without the life experience I could not cry out with recognition 'That's it in a nutshell!' The books and living complement each other. Nonetheless I heed the warning.

---

[7]You later commented that this was the first time that you had used such a form of address. You wrote how it showed 'how I appreciated you for your humanness, not as some expert who had all the answers'.

[8]On reflection, I realize that I could have benefited from cautioning myself against *urging* caution.

Fostering action

As you began to roam more freely through your own experience of 'Mistress Uncertainty', I offered you some highly specific questions framed as assignments. I offered you a pretty vague set of 'tasks' that you could pick and choose from, in an effort to find out what you 'made' of these kind of experiences. I could be accused in so doing of turning curiosity into plain old-fashioned nosiness, but I was interested to know what you 'found' in undertaking such tasks.

Many years ago, when I began to doubt the value of what went on within the consulting room (specifically), I encountered David Reynolds, who had written wisely (Reynolds, 1985):

> There is a myth in our culture that something magical occurs during an hour of psychotherapy ... Many people seem to believe that what happens during the golden hour is sufficiently powerful to colour the rest of the week. They seem to believe that the other 167 hours of the week have less effect than that one hour. Even some therapists agree. To succumb to this myth is to relegate the 167/168ths of life to meaninglessness. Life must be lived moment by moment. Each moment carries a message, a lesson for us. There are no golden hours, only ready people.

And so our sessions were more like rehearsals for the real-life stage. In that sense, your decision to call me 'coach' was apposite.

Towards the end of the therapy I began to notice how you were 'noticing' things more in your everyday life, and relating them to the whole of your experience. That seemed like a good time to focus on including discrete 'meditative' assignments as part of the 'working out' from the sessions in the clinic into the wider world of your experience. Most of my ideas about such assignments are influenced by David Reynolds (Reynolds, 1983, 1985). Although much of your reflection appeared to be philosophical in nature, it was important to anchor this in the more fundamental business of 'being' and 'doing'. Life still existed 'to be lived'. Reflection, however important, was no more than an image of how you had lived your life to date. And so I began to encourage you to extend your activities. Among the suggestions that I had developed from David Reynolds' work were:

- Dig, plant and care for a garden (although this could just as easily have been a potted plant)
- Write a journal of the sounds that you hear
- Give something away that you value to someone who can't repay you
- Give a name to a feeling that you have experienced, a feeling which has no name in English
- Keep a journal about what you have received from others, what you have returned to them, and what troubles you have caused during the day.

These tasks – all of which I had undertaken myself – I described simply as ways of 'extending yourself'. I hoped that they would provide opportunities for experiencing something of what you could or could not do. Clearly one can care for a plant, but this does not *mean* that the plant will thrive; we remain at the mercy of Mother Nature. Similarly, the tasks involving giving things away or naming un-named emotions offer the chance to step beyond the functional materialism of our everyday social world and enter a world of our own making. This may, ultimately, be the world where the *eternal truths* hold precedence (Kopp, 1974).

Funny, so much has been unpredictable and yet I find I am conforming to known patterns. For some time now I have been meaning to start guitar lessons. I decided this for several reasons and considered the best time would be when our work was almost done. So I smiled to read this morning that you suggest extending activities.

The bit about 'give away something valuable' got me thinking. Ever since I was introduced to Blake at university I have cherished 'the songs'. They have always been able to speak directly to me, though I wonder if I will ever truly understand all their meaning. Several times when I was working with C I tried to offer them as a tool in the therapeutic process – a way into my thoughts and feelings. He shunned my attempts to share books and music. I gave value to these things, and felt my offerings to be rejected and unvalued. I was interested in your questioning of what something is worth, and where does the value come from?[9] I placed great value on these things. At that stage it was a huge step to lay myself open (as I thought) in this way. Now I see from this point of view that these offerings had little value. Such important things to me would be just learning second-hand instead of living. I don't agree, but I see the point of view.

I remember when I gave him my brother's copy of Blake, he cried and cried. I was afraid. I didn't understand. Now I can read his letter from that time and understand he put a different value on that gift. He saw it as some sort of turning point in the relationship, I think. I gave him a spare copy of a book because I wanted him to read the book and hear what I was hearing in the words, but the value he placed on it was as an object that belonged to my beloved brother. I doubt he has ever read any of the poems.

Similarly, I tend to imbue situations with terror where none exists. When friends go on journeys, they always give me a full itinerary with flight numbers, departure and arrival times. In the past I have been maniacal about checking that flights arrive safely, or trains and buses get to their destinations without incident. There is nothing worse than knowing there has been a fatal accident and having to wait hours until

---

[9]I too was genuinely interested to know 'from where' the value came, that you found 'attached' to these things.

the police will issue IDs. This is foolish. I am trying now to let people go without giving me details. If anything does happen to someone I care about, I will find out soon enough. As my granny, who had a laundry list of her own, would say: 'What's afore ye will no ging by ye'. The trick is not to go looking for or expecting sadness, only to be ready to deal with it when it happens your way.

I note (in your writing) that you always refer to the patient as her. Is it only women who become strong enough/weak enough to do this work?

I appreciate it is difficult to establish an endpoint. Really that is because there is no such thing. I remember telling you once before that when I stopped evolving I would die. My experience of therapy is that it has brought me to an awareness of my evolution. Since the evolving is continuous, there is no endpoint. But of course our relationship must find a conclusion. How and when I can't answer. I gain from being with you, but I also know I wouldn't stop gaining from not being with you. The answer is probably that someone else needs you more. But I'm selfish!

Mutually selfish

Maybe the therapeutic relationship can only work if it is based on some kind of reasonable mutual selfishness. True, you had your own needs that required to be met. However I, like the other therapists you encountered, also had needs to be met, to maintain the balance of what might easily become a draining, one-sided relationship. I carefully crafted a structure for our 'conversations' that I hoped would be appropriate to meet your needs, but which also satisfied many of my ambitions to make sense of the whole business of therapy, if not also my developing role as a therapist. So in addition to employing some of the received wisdom from psychodynamic psychotherapy, person-centred therapy and cognitive behavioural therapy, I included metaphors, riddles and reflections from writers as diverse as the modern humanistic therapists and the ancient wisdom of Zen masters. I introduced these various 'alternatives', in part because I believed that such careful eclecticism would be of therapeutic benefit to you, but perhaps because these meditations on the core theme of therapy were inherently meaningful to me. I appreciated, however, that I was by no means alone in embracing such therapeutic flexibility:

> ... the dilemma is whether a therapist should practice as an ideological partisan or as an eclectic. The partisan (e.g. the psychoanalyst, the radical behaviourist, the reflective Rogerian) stays with the principles and techniques of a particular mode of therapy, whereas the eclectic uses techniques as they fit, regardless of theoretical purity. Accused of theoretical sloppiness, if not contradiction, the eclectic therapist is likely to take satisfaction and confidence from the precision of the technique-to-problem fit ... con-

trary to common sense and conventional wisdom, different therapies are not more effective with different problems.

(Lueger and Sheikh, 1989).

Having practised within many of the main schools of traditional 'Western' psychotherapy, I had come to appreciate that all psychotherapies ran the risk of becoming restricting ideologies. The 'school' or 'movement', with all its attendant rules and obligations, risks becoming a secular religion rather than a medium through which we all might gain access to the human truths of all our selves (Masson, 1985, 1989).

All forms of psychotherapy involve learning, although some are more explicit than others about this aim. I saw learning – for both you and me – as lying at the heart of the interaction, but unlike many forms of therapy this emphasis on learning lay closer to the surface of our relationship, even when what needed to be explored and learned from was abstract and elusive. And so we created an atmosphere of continuous learning, from one session to the next. This continuity was enhanced greatly by our mutual correspondence on various themes that had emerged from the sessions. Given your experience of other forms of therapy and clinical contact, which may have been less 'transparent' in communicating their aims and revealing the therapist's agenda, I emphasized the importance of sharing or pooling knowledge of 'what' needed to be done within a session.

Of course, like the other therapists you had encountered, I had my own therapeutic agenda. I wanted you to develop your awareness of how you constructed your own reality. I wanted to help you to make meaningful connections between what you thought (and believed) and how you felt about things that had happened in your life. In so doing, I was sharpening your focus not only on the nature and function of your distress, but also on what that distress might ultimately mean for you – and you alone.

This structure – because with hindsight it seemed to work – was a practical undertaking for both of us. You were cautious about 'yet another therapeutic relationship'. I was cautious about diving into waters that contained, as far as I was aware, who knew what? Consequently, the initial sessions involved putting you at ease, doing things that developed your trust in me and in the new therapeutic process. It needs saying that those early sessions also helped develop my confidence about the route that I was taking. I was working largely in the dark, feeling my way. To say that both therapist and patient are 'checking one another out' in those early stages is something of an understatement, for that simple phrase belies the complexity of what might be happening for both parties.

The intermediate stage focused again on doing something practical to address the distress that had first brought you to therapy. As you have described elsewhere, my approach appeared unconventional, since I was not wedded to any particular method but was curious, pragmatic and flexible. I was interested to know 'what worked for you', rather than to suggest that you employed something that had worked for someone else. This continued to develop the focus on the potential uniqueness of *your* experience. Such self-study ultimately provided you with some 'methods' to live with, and perhaps even to transcend your distress. My experience of your self-study was no less rewarding, helping me to hone my appreciation of what 'effective helpfulness' might be all about.

Finally, we sharpened the focus on how you might move out of this therapeutic context, taking your learning into the rest of your life. At the risk of sounding grandiose, this stage involved some kind of reconstruction of the 'self' – developing an appreciation of who Bobbie was – that was more philosophical (and flexible). On reflection, you seemed to see clearly the value of that stage.

I suppose what I'm really trying to say is that we always encourage in the therapeutic relationship a vision of the future, a vision of an independent person meeting the world with enthusiasm and confidence, ready to change and be changed.

No doubt many readers will argue that some other therapeutic approach – perhaps even one that I might risk dismissing as a 'therapeutic ideology' – might have proven just as effective, and also have been more efficient. However, the therapy that developed *is* the therapy that developed; there is no going back on that now. Maybe it was *exactly* the kind of therapy that needed to develop, given the nature of the two parties involved and all that we brought with us to the therapeutic encounter.

References

Barker, P. (1992). *Severe Depression: A Practitioner's Guide.* Chapman and Hall.

Barker, P. (1999). *The Philosophy and Practice of Psychiatric Nursing*, Preface. Churchill Livingstone.

Brenner, C. (1976). *Psychoanalytic Technique and Psychic Conflict.* International Universities Press.

Kopp, S. (1974). *If You meet the Buddha on the Road, Kill Him!* Sheldon Press.

Lueger, R. J. and Sheikh, A. A. (1989). The four forces of psychotherapy. In: *Healing East and West: Ancient Wisdom and Modern Psychology* (A. A. Sheikh and K. S. Sheikh, eds), pp. 103–38. John Wiley and Sons.

MacLaverty, B. (1998). *Grace Notes.* W. W. Norton

Malcolm, J. (1982). *Psychoanalysis: The Impossible Profession*, p. 25 and p. 37. Corgi Books.

Masson, J. (1985). *The Assault on Truth: Freud's suppression of the Seduction Theory.* Penguin.

Masson, J. (1989). *Against Therapy: Warning – Psychotherapy may be Hazardous to Your Mental Health.* Collins.

Moore, T. (1994). *Soulmates: Honouring the Mysteries of Love and Relationships*, p. 256. Element Books.

Reynolds, D. (1983). *Naikan Psychotherapy: Meditation for Self-Development.* University of Chicago Press.

Reynolds, D. (1985). *Playing Ball on Running Water*, p. 56. Sheldon Press.

Stevenson, W. H. (ed.) (1989) *The Poems of William Blake.* Longman.

Sullivan, H. S. (1953). *The Interpersonal Theory of Psychiatry.* W. W. Norton.

Watts, A. (1991). *The Essential Alan Watts*, p. 135. Celestial Arts.

Watts, A. (1993). *The Wisdom of Insecurity*, p. 74. Rider.

6

The promotion of growth and development

No individual will be judged by whether they come up to or fall short of some fixed result, but by the direction in which they are moving ... The process of growth, of improvement and progress, rather than the static outcome and result, becomes the significant thing. Not health as an end fixed once and for all, but the needed improvement in health – a continual process – is the end and good. The end is no longer a terminus or limit to be reached. It is the active process of transforming the existent situation. ... Growth itself is the only 'moral' end.

John Dewey (Munitz, 1979)

Introduction

I have always believed that therapy, given its 'healing' root, would involve some kind of 'growth' process. Of course growth has become something of a weasel word, and clearly means different things to different people. Since I held this belief about growth, albeit vaguely, long before I began to study and practise therapy, and indeed long before I read John Dewey, it must come from some general field of influence in my life rather than being a specific part of the therapeutic process itself. Looking back, however, it is clear that the therapeutic path I have taken reflects my pursuit of ways of reflecting, if not confirming, those original assumptions. I have sought ways of confirming my assumptions about the nature of growth in all our lives. The idea that all of us have the potential to grow imperceptibly 'forwards' in life made an uncommon kind of common sense to me. That said, I recall being urged all too often in childhood to 'grow up' – which implied a more rapid, dramatic and direct form of self-change than we are discussing here. Such motivation to somehow abandon childhood for a more 'mature' view of the universe risks turning us into jaded, dull and cynical adults. Instead, true maturity might involve maintaining our childlike innocence at the heart of adult selves; by retaining the simplicity of our child-self, we maintain our appreciation of the joys and the mysteries of life. For life can be an endless experiment in experience. Retaining such an experimental/experiential outlook on life, our child/adult understands Basho's (Basho, 1985) call:

> Look, children, hailstones!
> Let's rush out!

However, such casual usage of the vernacular did reinforce again the centrality of growth within the whole human project.

I don't recall us ever talking specifically about 'growth' within the sessions, but it was something that jumped the queue, so to speak, when we came to reflect on the process in considering the idea of this book. To what extent did I think you had 'grown' and, more importantly, what awareness of growth had you developed? So this chapter may well turn out to be another part of my efforts to reassure myself that my core beliefs and values – about people and life – are meaningful, not least in the context of your experience of therapy. I believe that the evidence of our therapy confirmed my assumptions about people and life, but the reader might well see the reverse case illustrated.

Feeling and being: the evidence of existence

For most people the process of psychotherapy is tied up inextricably with feelings and emotions. It was that abstract world of emotion that first prompted you to go seeking therapy, though even then you were not sure whether you were being led or being pushed in that particular direction.

Reflecting on those 'original' emotions, you wrote:

Towards the end of '86 there were a lot of bad stories on the go. It seemed men 'doing bad things to children' was in every paper you looked at, and on every TV and radio news bulletin. I couldn't get it out of my head. I couldn't deal with it.

It all began, I suppose, with Joseph and Mary, the first two people I ever felt really close to, cared about and loved by. They were also people who allowed me to return those feelings – something that I had only ever experienced with kids before. They used to make me feel like a part of their family. They even used to say that I was, which gave me the deepest sense of security I have ever experienced. It also gave me one of the greatest senses of loss when they no longer seemed able to give me so much.

We spent a lot of time together, and they found out quite a lot about me. I had never shared so much with anyone in my whole life before. The strange thing was, I never felt threatened by them. When I was feeling threatened I wanted to be with them, and they never pushed me where I couldn't go. I learned to be quite comfortable with them hugging me, and I got to like it once the first shock of them doing it, and in public too, went away. I never felt I was taking anything from them. It was more like they had so much to give, I was just getting some of what was going spare.

To cut a long story short, we were close for almost two years when things started to go wrong. They started to have some problems of their own, which at first I thought were a sign that I had done something wrong. Anyway, I started to feel uneasy in their home, stopped feeling part of the family, and my complete lack of understanding about what was happening made me feel horribly isolated. In the end I withdrew, and it has taken me years to come to terms with the relationship.

On top of the situation with Mary and Joseph, I was having the upheaval of 'camping' in one room of a new flat while joiners and plumbers ripped out and reconstructed the rest of it. Suffice to say, it all got to be too much for me.

One evening just a few days before Christmas, I had visited a colleague from work who was looking forward to his first Christmas with his new wife. Eric's mum was there, knitting a jumper for his sister in secret. They were really looking forward to the festivities, and all the talk was of a big family Christmas. We always used to have big family Christmases at our house, but since our family has been decimated it is just Mum and Dad and me, very conscious of the contrast. For a long time, Christmas stopped being a very happy time for me.

That night I just knew I was going to throw a wobbler, and I had to get out of Eric's house quickly and into a safe place. I was in such a hurry to get away, I fell the whole way down the stone steps from his upstairs flat to the ground floor. There was blood and grit everywhere, and all I remember is Eric picking me up and carrying me upstairs. Next thing, I came to with his Mum on her knees in the living room, tears pouring down her cheeks, cradling me in her lap. Eric's wife was sitting quietly beside us, and Eric was nowhere to be seen. He said later that his presence seemed to be upsetting me. They put me to bed in the spare room, and next morning I got a knock at 7.30 am and Eric comes in and puts his arms round me and says 'Bobbie, I had no idea you were so sad'. I panicked and wondered what on earth I'd been saying, and left quickly to go to work.

That night I went down to Eric's mum to apologize for my behaviour and try and find out what I'd said to her. A lot of it was about my siblings who had died. Eric's Mum had also got the negative message about my surviving brother, and I couldn't believe I ever said that in front of anyone. She started to cry again, but she said she wanted me to go and see somebody who could help.

And so you set off looking for help. First was a psychologist. That didn't work out, because he was far too direct for your liking. Then came the counsellor, who also didn't work out, and then came the female analyst. All tried to help, in their own quite different ways, but maybe they never got far enough with the bigger project, which was you developing your own capacity to help yourself. As Dewey put it, helping you to appreciate the direction in which you had been moving, unawares and unaided. Maybe that is the beginning and end of the therapeutic project – to help the person to develop an awareness of the change that is already taking place within her, and to harness that power.

Although the value and validity of Freudian psychology is now held greatly in doubt, culturally we have come to accept the significance of past experience as an influence on the present, and the idea that we need to 'go back' to retrieve the situation. We have also become hung up on an even more fixed and linear construction of our world and how we live it. We act often as if life is lived in stages – confirmed by Piaget's ideas about child development, and long ago in Shakespeare's 'ages of man'. Yet these are illusory 'stages'. If our lives *do* anything, they flow through us like a virtual ocean of experience. We *know* that we are alive, not so much by our reference to where we are at any stage in life, but by the discrete feelings we have about our more general state of *being*.

Whereas many people define their *selves* by reference to things 'outside' of themselves, people who come to therapy often possess an acute sense of their own being and how it *feels*. They recognize that this acute awareness of 'something' intangible separates them from the mass of their peers, many of whom appear only to drift through life almost like sleep-walkers, kept in line by the various social signals – like occupation, social status, peer relationships and so on. Often it is only the loss of one or more of these life markers that provokes a reflection on the age-old question – who exactly am I, and what am I doing here?

Many people who come to therapy have been exposed to some of the threats that the ocean of experience can offer. They may have been exposed to the human equivalent of storms and shipwreck that we now refer to, sanguinely, as traumatic stress. They may have been boarded, metaphorically, by pirates, and experienced a robbery of the self. Or they may have felt that they were drifting perilously towards some invisible rocks, or – perhaps even worse – were becalmed, like the Ancient Mariner, awaiting the fate decreed by his past misdeeds. These metaphors may be apposite, for most people rarely discuss their lived experience in the concrete, static language of mental illness, which assumes that people are either at fixed points in life, or possess equally fixed states within them. Instead most people talk like poets, lyrically expressing their *sense* of whatever it is that ails them, knowing that words are invariably inadequate but that words are all we have to communicate.

Although they are rarely aware of it, most people have already done a lot of vital work in 'living with' whatever it is that ails them. I have long been amazed that people in great emotional distress can even manage to make the necessary arrangements to attend the appointment. When you are, metaphorically, 'all at sea', organizing something as simple as attending for an appointment is no mean feat. I wonder how often I have forgotten that. At that first meeting, I looked for indications of what you might already be doing for yourself. As we now commonly say, 'if it ain't broke, don't fix it'.

That short extract from your journal about the circumstances that brought you to therapy showed just how hard you had worked to live with your past, and also to move beyond the limitations that your past had put on you. Joseph and Mary were your therapeutic ideal – accepting, giving and asking for nothing in return. A new experience for you, at least in terms of how these three human qualities were put together. But, as often happens, they found themselves no longer able to hold that position, and had to look after themselves. And so you were thrown headlong into a maelstrom that offered just the crisis you needed to provoke you into finding a professional analogue for Joseph and Mary.

Although therapists are loath to admit it, people generally find more support and resolution in ordinary relationships with wise and kind people than they do with therapists. The beauty of therapists is that, at least when they are working with you, they should be able to handle every kind of emotional experience you bring to them. They leave their personal egos at the door, so to speak, and adopt the professional's cloak of confidence. Friends like Mary and Joseph had no such safety net.

Feelings: the mentor within

As we have discussed in other chapters, our first encounter was pragmatic – I addressed what you brought with you. I didn't go 'looking' for anything. I had no 'therapeutic agenda'. I tried to begin with no preconceptions as to *what* might be the 'problem'. Similarly, I began with no preconceptions as to what might need to be done to address, and potentially to resolve, the problem. I assumed that you knew the nature of the problem and, by implication, knew what the resolution of the problem might *be* like. That approach seemed to work. In the very first session my rambling inquiries – I following you, rather than the reverse – seemed to lull you, and you fell into a deep trance[1] within which you revealed the great store of imagery that you were later to use more directly in responding to everyday crises.

On that first meeting, I felt that my pragmatic approach had again been

---

[1]On that first occasion I had no intention of *putting* you into a trance, but I had become aware over many years that a certain style of inquiry put people at their ease and helped them to open themselves to aspects of their experience that were normally beyond their awareness. When you *went* into the trance, I followed and, through gentle inquiry, helped you gain access to personal experiences that were remarkably 'self-reassuring'.

confirmed, at least for you, as appropriate. And so the therapeutic relationship continued, with me helping you to draw from your existing but largely hidden store of personal resources to 'live better' with whatever it was that ailed you[2].

However, during the early sessions you became aware of 'swinging' to and fro between the optimism that followed the session and quite different emotions that cropped up, apparently spontaneously. Like many people, you found the early sessions reassuring. Later in your journal you would record your frustration, wishing that I would 'just *make* my head fall off again, like that first time'. It was interesting that as you felt your 'head fall off', out came all sorts of vivid, positive imagery which, as you described it, lit up your face. The differences in Bobbie that already lay within you had begun to be revealed in the therapeutic process. The growing that had been going on, largely unnoticed, was now coming to the fore, and would become the main item on the therapeutic agenda. Although they could be disturbing and unnerving, your feelings were, as before, bringing you messages about the reality of your experience. In that sense, your emotions were always right, never wrong. They were your internal guide to the journey through life, and would act as guide and mentor to you throughout the therapeutic process.

Wednesday, October 7 11.00 pm

I don't know what I want to say, but I do want to talk to you so we'll just wait and see what pops out. I wish I could tell you I've extracted some great wisdom from thoughts and happenings in recent days, but I haven't – not yet, anyway.

Mostly I have just been feeling extreme, even when I tell myself to stop being like that because it's not right. I feel particularly bad at feeling so hacked off with you. I hope you aren't angry with me for that. That's all gone now, which I'm glad about, but what's so very perplexing is that I can no more explain how it went than how it came.

Do you think you can be too aware of feelings? I am often being told I don't have enough or am not aware of the ones I've got, but really I think that now I'm trying hard to understand and do this work with you properly, maybe I've just got too self absorbed. Maybe some things will work out okay for themselves in their own good time, with or without angst.

Three issues leapt from that short entry: your fear that I might judge you harshly; your driving desire to do things 'right'; and, perhaps most

---

[2]It is notable that at that first meeting I never sought to establish the *real* or *underlying* problem. For me, such experiences were simply other ways of re-presenting yourself. What you brought with you – or what brought you – to therapy on that particular day had to be the starting point. Where else could we have begun but at this new beginning, since within the context of my ocean of experience metaphor, every moment is a new beginning.

importantly, your growing realization that 'awareness of feelings' could be a bigger problem than the feelings themselves. These three issues were to dominate the developing therapy.

I began this chapter with an admission of what might be viewed by some therapists as an unrealistic belief in the 'rightness' of the person who had come in the guise of the patient. This 'optimistic' view of therapy is most strongly associated with Carl Rogers, so perhaps I need to say something about his thinking, since it certainly has helped me to develop my understanding of my own intuitive approach to therapy.

Rogers helped to shape a change in attitude towards the idea of the 'core' human being. The attitudinal set that underpinned the traditional therapy of Rogers' early days (he began to practise in 1928) could be described as 'humanely pessimistic'. Rogers noted that to the end of his life, Freud had believed that the negative influences of the *id* were inherently destructive and, in Karl Menninger's view, cast man as 'innately evil' (Rogers, 1956). Many took the view that Freud had inherited the tradition of St Augustine, through his belief that man was basically and fundamentally hostile, antisocial and carnal. By taking an oppositional – more optimistic – view, Rogers was seen, by some at least, to be the successor to Rousseau in assuming that everyone is a perfect being, since he comes from the hand of his Maker (as Rousseau believed). Rogers proffered an alternative view by suggesting that Freud and Calvin had more in common, especially in respect of the natural 'evil' of man.

Although I would not describe myself as a 'Rogerian'[3], these few lines from Rogers sum up elegantly my attitude towards therapy, which was reflected in our encounter (Kirschenbaum and Henderson, 1990):

> All individuals have within themselves the ability to guide their own lives in a manner that is both personally satisfying and socially constructive. In a particular type of helping relationship, we free the individuals to find their inner wisdom and confidence, and they will make increasingly healthier and more constructive choices.

That attitude appears to be the key distinction between the Freudian view of human nature and the person-centred approach. Rogers was followed by a wide range of other therapists, all emerging from the broad 'humanistic psychotherapy' school which he helped establish and all espousing the same 'unrealistic assumptions' that the patient had the capacity to heal her or himself. That said, Rogers himself admitted (Rogers, 1957) that although:

> clients (sic) can, to some degree, independently discover some of their denied or repressed feelings, they cannot on their own achieve full emo-

---

[3]Indeed, I could only describe my person-centred approach to therapy as 'personal', reflecting all the understandings and foibles of my own selfhood.

tional acceptance of these feelings. It is only in a caring relationship that these 'awful' feelings are first fully accepted by the therapist and then can be accepted by the client.

It was notable that you found just such a 'caring relationship' with Joseph and Mary. Had that relationship prospered, you might never have found the need for formal therapy. However, by the time you reached me your unsuccessful 'tour' through the other therapists appeared to have heightened your natural ambition to 'win through' by earnestly positive action; hence your desire to do the therapy 'right'. Those unsuccessful experiences had also, perhaps, sensitized you to the possibilities of therapist failure, if not outright rejection; hence your desire that I should not be offended by your failings. These two issues shared, arguably, the same historical space within you – functions of your Calvinistic upbringing[4]. However, the third issue you raised – your 'awareness' of the importance of the awareness of feelings – signalled the therapeutic moves that already were afoot within you; extensions of the therapeutic manoeuvres that characterized the session. I could hardly have said, there and then, 'don't worry, I don't get offended' or 'that's what I'm here for, to be offended'. Such comments would, however true, have appeared trite if not smug. Instead I probably continued with the style of inquiry that you found so irritating, but eventually unpicked for yourself, as I explored 'what (exactly) would be so bad about that, anyway?', seeking to establish further our conjoint understanding of what all of that might mean for you, there and then.

The examined life[5]

Our first encounter began as polite, tentative conversation. When we parted company we were still engaging in much the same conversation, but it had some special characteristics, which we might note here before moving on.

My assumption of your 'wisdom', which I suggested is close to Rogers faith[6] in humanity, has a much more ancient root. Socrates

---

[4]Which makes the reference to Freud's Calvinistic leanings all the more apposite.

[5]For Socrates, who suggested that 'the unexamined life is not worth living', the examination of life might result in *self-knowledge*. The knowledge to which he referred was not derived from reading a lot of books. Instead it meant such things as making the right kind of choices as a result of reflection, steering one's way (skilfully) through life's problems, crises, opportunities and options. This kind of *practical wisdom* is, arguably, what people intuitively come to therapy for. Increasingly, however, they are offered a diet of well-rehearsed 'scriptures' on how to live, or at least on how to resolve their problems, which require that they abandon the reflective uncertainty espoused by Socrates in favour of following the 'path to resolution' suggested by some theory or model of human conduct.

[6]It is worth noting that Rogers originally studied theology, and might have become a minister of religion had not he found religious doctrine offered, for him, a highly restrictive understanding of the 'meaning of life' (Rogers, 1961).

acknowledged that he was a 'midwife' of ideas, unable himself to give birth to wisdom, for in his view, ' I myself can bring nothing to light because there is no wisdom in me' (Taylor, 1953). Socrates asserted that people had ideas that were in a process of continual germination, and that his task was simply to help bring them out, as a midwife delivers a child. Although the concept of 'Socratic dialogue' is now frequently used within the psychotherapy literature, often this seems to mean a style of questioning by which the therapist encourages the patient to reveal the absurdity of his construction of present events (Beck *et al.*, 1980). For Socrates – and, much later, Rogers – this was not a disingenuous trick; rather it was an honest acknowledgement that one person can have no true knowledge of another person's thinking and the world of experience to which it relates. It follows that one way to approach this state of ignorance is to learn from the person through helping them to clarify and give birth to the meanings of their situation.

So when Socrates talked of his *dialectic*, he did not mean this in the grand sense intended by Hegel and Marx when they talked of the *patterns* or laws of history. Instead, Socrates meant the critical examination of a person's ideas, opinions and beliefs through conversation (*dialektike*) or *dialogue*.

At the outset, I had no idea of the true nature of your problem, far less what were your therapeutic needs. By that I mean that although I knew that the analyst had recommended that 'you needed to learn to relax', I had no idea that this was what you needed (as opposed what she needed) to further the analysis. More importantly, I had no reason to believe that your 'need' might have changed as you transferred from working with the analyst to working with me. Uncertainty was the one thing of which I was certain. I was fairly certain that you too would be uncertain and, paradoxically, out of our conjoint uncertainty might grow awareness.

Sunday, July 26 7.10 pm

You really started something asking me to notice changes. Once you get into it, it's a never-ending task. I figure that is exactly what it is, because what we are looking at together is the evolution of me, and evolution never ends. When I stop evolving, I will be dead. Have I got it right?

The thing I notice about evolution is, you can't stop it even when you want to. That's what I notice about my friendships. Sometimes when you feel things are changing, but maybe you want to stay close and stem the drifting away feeling, well you can't. Even noticing that's happening changes it, and you can't get back to where you think you were happy because nobody is standing still. Sometimes the best bit is much later, when you can look back and say, 'well, I'm glad I had that friendship, but I'm glad too it changed or maybe I wouldn't have found this other one'. Don't you think that if we try to hold on to things and stop things changing, we do die a bit, because we limit ourselves and our ability to be open to new experiences? Well that's how it seems to me anyway.

This pattern of thinking had been developing over the day, as you noted, because you had visited Mary and Joseph, 'the first two people I have ever felt really close to, cared about and loved by'. You continued:

At that time Joseph and Mary's three children were all still very young, and the family didn't have a car. I was the only one in the {families of disabled children} group who didn't have a family of my own to look after, so I felt it was up to me to arrange my life around their needs for the time their daughter was ill. In the beginning they were just people from the group who needed helping out, but over those two months we got very close.

In the end there was nothing anybody could do for the wee girl, and she died just before 11 o'clock in the morning.

The Browns are committed Catholics and I am a committed atheist. One of the things that really got to me was that, knowing I would be clueless, Joseph phoned me the day before the Reception of the Remains and explained to me all that would happen that night and at the funeral the following day. He didn't want me to go in unprepared, but they did want me to be there. I just couldn't get over the fact that in the middle of all their sadness they were thinking about how I would feel, and were trying to help me cope. It was a very sad time but it was a very special time too, and to be honest I will be forever glad to have had the experience.

Although that relationship was eventually to grow difficult, you became aware then of its eternal importance, if you like. Maybe that is one of the strangest secrets about life; that everything that ever happens to us we get to keep, whether good or ill. Even when things happen to change our view of those events – historically speaking, as we look back on them – they still endure. Experience may be fleeting, but the recall of experience can last throughout a lifetime. And here in the bosom of this family's grief you found the meaning of acceptance and compassionate caring. True, you might have expected this from any number of other people, but it was the Browns who *first* offered that to you. The special bitter-sweet nature of the occasion was left with you and, notwithstanding what happened thereafter, your experience of friendship at the hands and hearts of the Browns does seem like something worth being eternally grateful for.

Perhaps what you 'noticed' about your relationship with the Browns was the beginning of your encounter with 'Mistress Uncertainty', as you sensed the evolutionary and continually shifting nature of our everyday experience.

Within you – without you: the gaining of wisdom

Soon you began to 'see' versions of your own dilemma enacted on the life stage of people with quite different experiences – at least in terms of the detail of the script. This suggested to me that you were beginning to clarify what you might *really* need, to deal with these recurrent, troubling emotions; contrasting this, perhaps, with what you had experienced to date. And with that awareness of yourself in the reflection of some distant 'other' came a feeling of guilt.

Wednesday, August 19 11.40 pm

Dear Coach,

I read an article today which makes me feel fierce and frustrated. It's about a guy who survived the Piper Alpha inferno, who was banged up in gaol for cannabis offences. He said he took the drug to blot out the horror of the rig blast, but he still got 18 months. Could you do anything for a bloke like that? If ever there was a case for therapy as opposed to punishment, this is surely it. Okay, I accept that in an ideal world everybody would get the services they require whatever the cost, but we're not on that planet. But how do you decide who gets a slice of the pie? It can't be right that this guy gets shut in a cell, where isolation will surely only exacerbate his problems and give more free time for his nightmares, while I'm getting so many hours of professional time when, as you yourself admitted, I'm not sick[7].

I can't even begin to imagine the sort of disturbances the Piper men endure. I can still recall in minute detail the men and the families I visited in the days immediately following the disaster. If it haunts me, what can it be like for the men who were actually there?

I remember some months after the blast going back to speak to a scaffolder I'd spoken to on the Saturday after the inferno. He was virtually housebound, and told me he didn't like the phone to ring because it was the outside world coming into the safety of his own living room. All that guy had been offered by way of help was a social worker visiting once a week. As the scaffolder said, what did he have in common with a middle class social worker who liked to drink tea?

---

[7]Early on in the conversation (dialectic) you had asked me if I thought you were 'sick' or 'mentally ill'. Since these are medical concepts I am fairly confident that I said only that these were not meaningful for me. However, for what it's worth, all distress is relative, whatever it is called. You and the Piper Alpha survivor may have had a lot in common in terms of human distress. Professional constructs – such as mentally ill, disordered, sick – serve only to confuse the laity, as Shaw first sagely observed.

> *I have read your own bit in your book (Barker, 1992), and it seems like a lot of common sense to me. Also I get the feeling that I am 'reinventing the wheel'. It seems that things I have discovered and worked out for myself are already written down in books. I feel quite cheated of what I thought were my own small successes. Even that simple thing about making yourself do chores before you get involved in good stuff has an official name. A book told me it's called 'delay of gratification'. Well, I might not have the fancy jargon, but what I worked out boiled down to the same thing, didn't it?*

I have no idea how empathetic you were before you began to 'notice' things within the reflective process, but here you express a powerful, indeed indignant, form of empathy. Maybe the plight of the Piper Alpha men helped you to view something of your own situation.

The reflective process, which Socrates would definitely have called an 'examination', is also bearing fruit. You are becoming wiser. Indeed, Socrates would have deemed this a true form of knowledge, a *practical wisdom* – for you found it within the examination of your lived experience. You are, of course, not dealing with any kind of tangible reality that can easily be described as a 'sickness' or 'not-a-sickness'. Rather, you are dealing with some of the intangibles of your own experience. The philosopher would describe this as ' the Truth of Being' (*aletheia*), which comes through a direct or immediate 'disclosure'; not through reading about it, or being told of this 'truth'.

> Its like coming out of a dark and tangled mass of buildings and winding streets, and suddenly seeing in full light the expanse of the ocean before you. There it is! You see it. It's right before your eyes, directly and immediately. It is 'lit up' for you. (Barker, 1992)

It is not surprising that you find that others have 'found' similar bits of wisdom before you, or at least have named something similar, as part of their own process of saying 'I was here'. What Bobbie found was her own version of the Truth and, as the movie credits frequently acknowledge, any resemblance to persons living or dead is entirely coincidental!

The emotional meaning of distress

Gradually you began to feel stronger, more confident – both human qualities that Socrates believed would be 'lit up' by the reflective process. However, ignorance can serve an important function too, even as it applies its emotional pressure. Enlightenment can have its drawbacks.

Monday, September 24 12.20 am

Dear Coach,

My feeling stronger has risks too. Now, looking back, I think I was holding on to my weakness because 'getting better' would mean I was out on my own. Very risky. Getting my confidence back, starting to deal with things, makes that seem imminent. That is scary. I think what's good is that I accept that. I'm not sure what to do about the scary bit, but I know I don't want to go back to the 'safety' of stagnation. I'm opting for the unknown, and taking a bet that's a risk worth taking.

Here you take the 'leap of faith', which you discuss in Chapter 7. The risks are obvious to you, but this is no rational, reasoning process. Rather, you are doing what needs to be done and, in terms of the ocean of experience, you are 'taking the plunge'.

Friday, September 28 8.00 pm

Dear Coach,

I thought I would want to talk to you about John, but I don't really. I thought I'd take a drive to the tree, which is still bared of the bark where he crashed into the trunk, but I don't really want to do that. The tree still bears the scars, but the land all round about it has been developed and a house has been built on the ground next to the burn where he drowned. It's ten years tonight since he didn't come home, and I really didn't think I felt anything anymore but I just started to cry. I don't know why. I felt a bit guilty today because today didn't feel any different to any other day, and somehow you feel it should, because how can someone have been that important to you and you don't feel anything anymore? For a long time I missed him so much it was a real, physical pain – well, that's what it felt like. For a lot of time in the very beginning I used to forget completely that he'd gone. I remember buying a jumper for his Christmas, then having to take it back because I remembered he wouldn't be home for Christmas. It was easy to forget he'd gone, because his death didn't make any change to the routine of my everyday life. I was already out living on my own, and he had been away at university for a year before he was killed, so I was used to our everyday lives being separate. But every so often I'd catch myself 'seeing' him in the street, and then get upset when I realized it was somebody else who had fair red hair, or a similar way of walking, or something else that made me think of him. Now I don't have intrusive thoughts about him. I think about him when I want to think about him, and it really doesn't hurt like a pain anymore. It just shows you can get used to absolutely anything – except at Christmas.
It's just the ordinary things that make you feel sad. A girlfriend at work

couldn't wait to tell me the other day she was an auntie again. Her sister had had another baby. I sometimes think how many real nephews and nieces I would have if I had surviving sibling relationships. Lots of kids call me auntie, but I wonder if it would be different if there were blood ties. It's a silly thing to wonder, because I'll never find out now.

Sorry, but I'm not being very positive today. It'll pass. I've actually got this whole date thing sussed. Since I got to know Derek, I've decided not to think of September 28 as the day John died but as the day Derek was born. Last year and the year before I really enjoyed the day because I was at his birthday party. He was supposed to be going to the Transport Museum in Glasgow with his daddy tomorrow for a birthday treat, but Bob has to work. The wee man was so disappointed his dad arranged to take him this afternoon instead, and the party for the rest of the boys and me will be tomorrow. I told him he would get my presents then, because I knew he would be dead beat by the time he got back tonight. It would have felt better tonight if I'd had cuddles from the boys today.

I don't know what I want today really. I don't really want to do this. I don't want to watch TV, can't concentrate on a book, and hate the feeling I've just given up and given in. I'm going, because if I keep this up I'll hate you too for nothing.

This was a poignant entry, for we had never discussed John – at least not directly. You had always kept to allusions, which was clearly the territory you needed to map. I felt the sadness, but I knew that what you had been feeling was a quite different order of sadness, tied as it was to all other sorts of tentative and fragile relationships. The ship of life needs often to steer a tricky course.

The simple act of committing these thoughts, and the feelings to which they were inextricably connected, seemed like a critical stage in the proceedings. Therapists often use all sorts of devices to chart 'therapeutic progress' or 'change'. Often these only measure the extent to which the patient is complying with her agenda, to desist from complaining or to achieve the kind of wisdom known already, too well, by the therapist. If you had asked me directly how it was going, up until that point I would probably have said 'fine', or something equally vague. When I read your journal entry, I knew that you had stretched yourself way beyond the boundary you had crossed previously with Mary and Joseph. This entry touched my heart, which is always the best arbiter of human activity.

Journey or pilgrimage?

Perhaps you too appreciated how far you had travelled. For the next entry began in a quite different, contemplative mood. You knew that you were increasingly 'out on your own', without the proverbial parachute.

After many years spent dealing, very silently, with your problems, the tearful empathy of Eric's mother had nudged you onto the therapy path. The search for a sustainable therapeutic relationship, within which you had the space to grow at your own pace, turned that search into something more like a journey. The true nature of that journey became clearer as you began to develop the simple yet elusive capability for emotional equilibrium into something closer to an acceptance of yourself and others – warts and all.

The pace you originally set was vigorous. Time was, invariably, of the essence. But over time the changes you noticed flashed and flickered, seeming to come and go. Progress down that path appeared erratic, and at times you felt that you were straying if not actually doubling back.

But things were changing. You were covering new ground, although all of it was, in the personal sense, old territory. You were reading aloud from your back pages. No mean feat, given that for so long you had tried to keep the book shut.

The nature of the relationship with me was changing too, albeit slowly. This is shown eloquently in the naming of names. At first, the address was 'Doctor' – a signal of hoped-for knowledge, if not wisdom, but also a means of keeping me at a professional distance. Soon, as the nature of our working relationship became clearer, I became 'coach', suggesting a kind of closeness, but also a lightness of touch. If I had ever played the game at which you were trying to become more proficient, it was a long time ago, and I could afford to be casual about the demands of the training and forgetful of the pressure that hope can apply. In time you were to leave this coaching territory also, as you began to appreciate, perhaps, that if the gains you were making were in any way akin to sporting prowess, this was a game without end. As you began to see the end of the path in sight, you finally twigged that I too was on this path, and so we began to walk side by side until the fork in the road was to separate us.

October 6 1992 8.20 am

Dear Fellow Pilgrim,

I was lying in bed in that place somewhere between sleep and full wide awakeness when the mind wanders, and I thought, 'better get up and write all this down'.

I was feeling concerned about all the things I haven't done in therapy, and very concerned that my brave speech about ending a couple of days ago was just that – a brave speech.

But don't worry, I've decided I'm not regressing – just making sure I've packed a mac! It's absolutely pishing down outside. I wouldn't go out in it if I didn't have to, unless I had a waterproof. Well I think that's what's happening to me in therapy. I want to make sure I'm properly prepared, and I've packed what I need before I set off.

While I was lying in bed, I was thinking about things I've yet to tackle with you: I felt I would regret setting out without doing work on these things. I know therapy could be never-ending, and you have to decide on an endpoint, but it concerns me that all this work will go to waste and I'll fall off the mountain because I didn't pack enough crampons or skipped on the altitude training. I feel that if I don't tackle these things they might well prove difficult when I start the lone assault, if only because I know I skimped on the preparation. I'll know I could've done more, and will be dogged by doubts of whether I've done enough to get by. I'm not a 50 per cent person. I don't want to do just enough to get a pass rate, if you can ever know what that is. I want to do well.

I'm sure this is not just a case of dragging it out some more, to put off the evil moment of going. I did consider that, but it's not the case. The way I looked at it was that the map showed several ways to get to the base of the mountain. It was hard to decide which route to take – the straightest route, or one of the routes through villages. It was impossible to decide which would be the quickest route. The straightest route had some very rough terrain that would make the passage slow, but a route through the villages mightn't be fast either, stopping to speak to people and giving a hand with the chores. It's an impossible decision, with too many unknown variables. So what does anybody do, faced with a choice like that? He makes the choice on the basis of the best available information, and does what feels right for him. So you might think I'm taking a little detour here, staying in the foothills longer than necessary, but I believe I am just making extra sure my backpack's got everything I'll need – a proper reassurance for the lone assault. Take care of the things you can, and you'll be better able to face the unknown. What do you think? But this is such an inexact science. I could equally argue that an athlete could be overtrained, that I could pack too much unnecessary clutter in my rucksack. At the end of the day you do your own thing, pick the therapist who says things you want to hear. Am I just taking the easy way? Can we ever really know the answer to that? Now where's that laundry list[8]!

You were referring to the list of 'unfinished business' that you wanted to add to the therapeutic agenda before we closed the book on therapy. Your insomnia certainly gave you a good time for reflection. I wonder to what extent what you eventually committed to paper was like the thoughts that had been running through your wandering mind. I have a hunch that the simple act of writing, like talking aloud as opposed to listening to the conversations in your head, results in that state we have elsewhere called re-authoring. The discipline of writing requires some editing. It also slows up the process, imposing a structure on that often scatterbrained thoughtfulness. It seems clear that the conversation you had, first with

---

[8]A reference to Sheldon Kopp (1974).

yourself and then with me (in the abstract), resulted in you answering –
to a large extent – some of the questions you had posed in the beginning.
This became clearer the next day.

Monday, October 7 11.50 am

I think Joyce McMillan (the Scotland on Sunday *columnist) has been
reading Sheldon Kopp. Or is it just that people who set out to discover
their world find a common language? Her description of the Royal
Dilemma was pure Kopp:*

> … getting married is never an answer, only a new set of questions …
> Diana's obvious suffering in her marriage, and Fergie's spirited flight from
> hers, will say more to millions of young women about the fallibility of mar-
> riage as a 'solution', and THE COMPLEXITY AND LONELINESS OF
> EACH INDIVIDUAL'S ROAD TO HAPPINESS (Bobbie's original empha-
> sis), than decades of feminist proselytising.

This was a very short note, but one full of gusto. You clearly heard a res-
onating echo of your own journey towards resolution. Was this the day
that you first realized that you already had all the answers you might
need? Or was this the day when you realized that 'solutions' that lay
'outside' would always be inadequate? Or was this the day that you
simply became more philosophical about the whole undertaking?

Just over two weeks later, you began to re-author some of your most powerful emotions – or at least some of the stories from your back pages,
which had long been dogging you, if not haunting you.

Dear Phil[9],

*I've got a reframe[10] for you. I've been working on it a long time – long
before I knew it was a reframe. You know you sometimes ask me how I
would like things to be in the future? Well when I used to go and see the
counsellor, my objective was to get to a point where I could have an ordinary relationship with my brother. How I imagined it was, I would be
really laid back and just ordinary around him. I figured that you needed
to have something you did together, on a fairly regular basis, to build a
relationship. So I decided I would learn to play darts and drink beer, and
maybe once a week we would meet up on neutral ground in a pub somewhere, and we would just be together like normal brothers and sisters.
That's how I really thought it would be. That's what I thought needed to*

---

[9]This familiarity was, perhaps, further evidence of how you were easing yourself out of the therapeutic relationship – finding confidence *in* yourself and your own feet.
[10]Evidence of your private study of the therapy literature.

happen for me to be straightened out and to make things equal between us.

Now I don't think this is what needs to happen and, more than that, I don't even want that to happen. He hasn't spoken more than ten words to me in as many years, so there's not a lot there to build on. Similarly, it doesn't make us equal if I try and change myself into something I'm not (a beer-drinking darts player) just to meet him on his ground. And, apart from a relationship requiring contributions from both sides, who says he wants me to meet him on his ground, or that he wants me to change, or that he gives a shit what I think or want, or even what he thinks and wants?

This reads like a pretty powerful 'reframe'. Clearly, you have shifted your position in relation to your (older) brother. Maybe this suggests that you have shifted your position in relation to yourself.

And, so you continued:

I have reframed a lot of bits about him, and I could probably do some more if my folks would give me the information I need to do it with. However, what I've done has been more or less by accident. For instance, I never could understand why, when he was always such a bad boy as a child, my parents always seemed to love him so much, repaying his badness with special toys. All the times the police would come to the house and me and the babies would hide under the dining-room table, and he still got a brand new racing bike. I never got a bike 'til I was eleven, when a woman took me under her wing and got one from the scrapper's and painted it for me. It was the only bike I ever had 'til I was old enough to buy my own. When he was getting his first two-wheeler I was supposed to get his old trike, but he drove it into the kerb so hard, so many times until it was so bent out of shape he stopped because he knew he'd ruined it and I wouldn't get it. He did some really evil things. I remember when I was in Primary Two, my class was on the stage singing in front of the whole school at assembly and I was taken out, right in front of everybody, and I didn't know why. When I got to the head teacher's, my mum was there with the police. Her engagement ring had been stolen from the mantelpiece in our house that morning. It turned out it was him and his friend who took it just before they left for school.

I always thought my granny was the worst one, though; my mother's mum. He did terrible things to her, and yet I always knew she adored him and would say my dad was too hard on him. My brother and I would be sent to stay with her for the summer, and she always made a difference between us – not in the things she gave us and did for us, but just how much she liked us. He had stolen lots of money from her (and I am not talking sixpences), but it wasn't until she got in a big mess not being able to pay a bill that my aunt found out and made her go to the police. But it seemed like every time he kicked Mum or Granny in the face, they kept

going back for more. It got to the stage I lost all respect for them over it.
I simply didn't understand it.

Sometime around the end of last year I began to work out something
of what was going on. My friend Bernard was talking to me about his
National Service. My dad did his in Germany too. It clicked that I was
born the year after he came home. He was in Germany two years, so I
realized he would have missed my brother as a baby. I could work out
that a kid on his own with his Mum for two years would resent a strange
man coming into the house, and it would be a strain for Dad coming back
and trying to fit into a totally changed domestic situation. Also, my
Granny was widowed in the war and had to bring up a young family on
her own. He was her only grandchild, and a boy at that. I bet he was
spoiled rotten when Dad was away, and I'll bet there were some bobby
dazzler fights and huffed silences between Dad and Granny about
methods of child-rearing once Dad was home. I think now my Dad was
probably always trying to make up to him for not being there in the begin-
ning.

I remember wanting to check all this out with my Mum, but she would-
n't discuss it. One thing she did tell me, though; when I asked when Dad
did National Service and how old was Henry when he went, she said he
got a two-week extension until the baby was born, then he had to leave
for Germany the day after Henry arrived. It made a lot of things more
understandable for me. Then imagine how Henry must have felt. He was
just about getting used to having a strange man in the house when I
arrived. In all the photographs we have, he is never smiling. He always
looks like he wants to punch someone in the face.

Also, I realize now he is dyslexic, but no one had ever heard of that
when we were going to school. I just remember Mum standing on a chair
screaming for them to stop, and Dad and Henry rolling around the
kitchen floor laying into each other. It was all because Dad had checked
his homework and he went berserk because at 14 he had got his bs and
ds round the wrong way. Now I know that's a classic sign of dyslexia, but
then I just thought he was born without brains. School must have been
torture.

Some things just can't be repaired, but you can find better explana-
tions for yourself. That's reframing, eh?

I've got another reframe about Henry on the night after my other
brother died, but I'm too whacked. I'll tell you about that some other
time.

It is a great privilege being a therapist. This privilege is not about being
privy to all sorts of skeletons and secrets, which is a privilege in itself,
but rather in being a kind of spectator at someone's passing out parade
and feeling that one had some kind of a hand in it. I think that was what
Socrates meant about being a 'midwife'. This story is manifestly about
you trying to 'see' your brother through a different pair of eyes, or setting

him in a different context, as the notion of the reframe suggests – literally putting a different frame of reference around the information you already have about him. However, it also can be read as a vehicle for seeing life through different eyes. The journey you have been taking doesn't lead anywhere, except possibly back home. As the Celts would say, the journey always leads back home, to the Sacred Centre.

Perhaps you are becoming aware that your story, which you have always tended to 'read' from only one perspective, is open to several possible readings. The question *who* is Bobbie? can be at one and the same time an impossible question to answer, *and* one that offers limitless possibilities. We could say that there are countless ways in which we might re-present ourselves – as you did with the story of Henry. However, *what* it is that you seek to re-present just *is*, and is not open to being re-presented.

I read that elegant reframe of the story of Henry as a clear sign that you were opening out to the infinite possibilities of your own personal universe. Many therapies seek to 'explain' how people became this way or that. If it is not a function of some deeply buried childhood events, it is a function of dysfunctional thinking, which also may have been developed in childhood. Many of these theories can be read, sanguinely, as no more than attempts at immortality by the theorists who framed them; expressing their own need to explain others, and perhaps – therefore – themselves. Perhaps the search for general 'explanations' is futile, since people like you can clearly arrive at your own, particular explanations.

These final musings from your journal suggest how far you had actually travelled. You would probably say that your were far from 'completed' or 'whole'. I might well say, 'join the club'.

A quick look over the shoulder

This chapter has emphasized the vagaries of growth and development – a process of becoming, rather than a ticket to any particular destination. All this talk of growth can easily be dismissed as a 'new-age' perspective on therapy, but I think that all it shows is that the pursuit of wholeness, the resolution of problems or – worse – their elimination, is a futile pursuit. People learn to live with uncertainty, or they seek solace in various systems that effectively deny the fickle nature of our everyday reality. I think that your evolution from someone with fairly concrete perspectives on life into someone who was willing to be more philosophical is shown in this short extract from our correspondence following the end of therapy.

It's difficult for me to decide where to usefully start the story of my experience of therapy. The way I behaved and the way I thought at the beginning of my therapeutic relationship with Phil (I always called him Dr

Barker in the early days) was different from the way I behave and the way I think now, even when reacting to similar stimuli. Similarly, the way I behaved and the way I thought was in constant change during therapy. So it seems to me I will have to think my present self into the memory of a particular self along the way to make any accurate kind of assessment of what was helpful in treatment and what was not. The sort of free-ranging exploration that went on during the latter stages of therapy would have been unworkable in the early stages.

I am conscious that I use the word helpful now, when in the beginnings of therapy I was obsessed with what was 'right' and what was 'wrong'. Again, what was 'right' for me at one stage wouldn't necessarily be 'right' for me three months down the line. All I know for sure is that at particular stages, particular approaches and particular suggestions were helpful.

I would feel hard-pressed to put my finger on any specific approaches that I thought had effected some of the gains that you allude to. Change involves a much bigger system of events, and certainly cannot be attributed to the effects of any one thing, as if you had been knocked forward like a billiard ball.

Indeed, the changes that for me were most significant involved changes in perspective. You shifted your position on so many things. Indeed, you shifted from the black-and-white thinking of right-versus-wrong that characterized your initial attitude set, to accepting a range of possibilities. Some might see that as a pretty remarkable shift, on its own.

In terms of your original emotional disturbance, it is not clear if this 'went' somewhere, or if you adjusted your consciousness of it. Certainly you became much more appreciative of what was happening outside of yourself, and also of the myriad meanings of all that, which might have been read as a reflection of the myriad meanings of you yourself. Alan Watts seemed to describe this neatly (Watts, 1997a):

> One of the highest pleasures is to be more or less unconscious of one's own existence, to be absorbed in interesting sights, sounds, places, and people. Conversely, one of the greatest pains is to be self-conscious, to feel unabsorbed and cut off from the community and the surrounding world.

And as you noted, such self-consciousness and the sense of being cut off from the outside world *is* the essence of mental illness.

Certainly, you seemed to 'find' yourself by getting 'lost' in all manner of things – from brushing your teeth to just *being* with people. Of course, the world outside of ourselves is fragile and fickle, and ultimately penalizes us. Again, as Watts sagely noted (Watts, 1997b):

> We seem to be like flies caught in honey. Because life is sweet we don't want to give it up, and yet the more we become involved in it, the more we

are trapped, limited and frustrated. We love it and hate it at the same time. We fall in love with people and possessions only to be tortured by anxiety for them. The conflict is not only between ourselves and the surrounding universe; it is between ourselves and ourselves. For intractable nature is both around us and within us. The exasperating 'life' which is at once lovable and perishable, pleasant and painful, a blessing and a curse, is also the life of our own bodies.

Watts appreciated only too well the search for certainty in an uncertain universe, for he too had been a seeker. When he came to consider how any of us might experience life 'as something other than a honey trap in which we are the struggling flies', he clarified for himself – and ultimately for the rest of us – the fundamental nature of that insecurity (Watts, 1997c):

> How are we to find security and peace of mind in a world whose very nature is insecurity? All these questions demand a method and a course of action. At the same time, all of them show that the problem has not been understood. We do not need action – yet. We need more light.

The idea of solving a problem implies finding out what to *do* about it. However, it also implies understanding it, which is perhaps where the 'finding out' comes into it. When we try to *do* something about a problem without really understanding it, this may be like trying to 'clear away darkness by thrusting it aside with your hands. When light is brought, the darkness vanishes at once' (Watts, 1997c). The simplest explanation of what 'happened' in the therapeutic process that took place between us was that both of us brought some light to bear on the situation. It was not simply you who felt in some way illuminated by the proceedings. The illumination that I discovered is another aspect of the privilege that I referred to earlier.

So, the question remains – have you grown, or have you simply shifted your position? Does the one merely betray the significance of the other? It certainly seems as if you have moved – and significantly so. You appear to have been involved in the *active process of transforming you existent situation,* as John Dewey put it, so long ago. His words seem very apposite today, in these 'new age' times, if only because they illustrate that the need to come to terms with ourselves and our experiences ultimately requires us to stretch our concept of ourselves beyond our 'existent situation'. That appears to be not so much a 'new-age' as a very 'old-age' project indeed. However, in the final analysis only you can judge whether or not you have come to terms with anything, far less grown or transformed your situation.

References

Barker, P. (1992). *Severe Depression: A Practitioner's Guide*. Chapman and Hall.

Basho, M. (1985) *On Love and Barley: Haiku of Basho*, (translator, L. Stryk). Penguin.

Beck, A. T., Rush, A. J., Shaw, B. F. and Emery, G. (1980). *Cognitive Therapy of Depression*. John Wiley and Sons.

Kirschenbaum, H. and Henderson, V. L. (eds) (1990). *The Carl Rogers Reader*, p. xiv. Constable.

Kopp, S. (1974). *If You meet the Buddha on the Road, Kill Him!* Sheldon Press.

Munitz, M. K. (1979). *The Ways of Philosophy*. Collier Macmillan.

Rogers, C. (1957). A note on 'the nature of man'. *J. Cons. Psychology*, **4(3)**, 199–203.

Rogers, C. (1961). *On Becoming a Person*, pp. 7–8. Houghton Mifflin.

Taylor, A. E. (1953). *Socrates*. Anchor Books, Doubleday.

Watts, A. (1997a). *The Wisdom of Insecurity*, p. 109. Rider.

Watts, A. (1997b). *The Wisdom of Insecurity*, p. 37. Rider.

Watts, A. (1997c). *The Wisdom of Insecurity*, p. 69. Rider.

7

The leap of faith

Be a lamp unto yourself. Be your own confidence. Hold on to the truth within yourself, as to the only truth.

Buddha

Risk taking

Although I spent most of my time trying to establish what you needed, and in particular *where* you needed to go, I was not averse to pointing out things on our journey together. In that sense, the nature of our therapeutic relationship differed markedly from that which you had experienced first (briefly) with the psychologist, then in a more focused sense with the counsellor and the analyst. I could say that my approach was more pragmatic, more eclectic in its introduction of ideas and influences from different 'schools' of therapy. However, although I don't know what was in the hearts and minds of those three other professionals, I know what was in mine. I was aware that I was asking you to take some very significant risks with yourself, and it was my responsibility to ensure that you were as aware as you could be of what you were letting yourself in for, if not what you were encountering. Your reflections on your whole experience of therapy appeared to reinforce the importance of that central fact.

I made two different 'leaps of faith' during therapy. The first was in desperation, coming from a feeling I had run out of options but had to try something, and whatever I was about to pitch into seemed like the only option available. The second 'leap' came from trust in another. This is the leap you make when you don't know where you are being taken, but you have confidence it is to a better place, a more exciting place, a place that breeds better options and where you have choice.

I made a leap of faith when I went to see the counsellor. That was the first kind of leap – made in desperation; a 'back to the wall' option.

Going to my GP was the next 'leap of faith', another last ditch option when I knew I wasn't coping and the symptoms were becoming more disabling. Actually, it wasn't a leap of faith, more of a step. I knew the GP wasn't going to be the person who would provide therapy, but just the link to the therapist. This knowledge affected my approach to the meeting and what I said. The meeting went amazingly well due solely to the fact I had the good fortune to be seen by a very astute lady. I had insisted on seeing a woman, and she picked up a lot from the little that was said and reassured me that I could be helped by someone who would be able to give me the time I needed. It would have been inappropriate to leap in and put my faith in the GP, and I knew her function was not to help me directly. In the current jargon, I suppose she was the 'enabler'.

But here's where it gets difficult for an ordinary Joe like me. When I went for my first psychiatric appointment, I thought I was about to make a leap of faith. It was certainly difficult trying to prepare myself for that first appointment. I didn't realize I was just going for an 'assessment', although the psychiatrist did make it quite clear once I was with her that she wouldn't be treating me, but would only be making a referral. That made it very difficult, and I pulled back. She must have had difficulty assessing what the problem was, because I certainly had difficulty responding to her, knowing that it would all have to be gone through again with another professional. I don't know what the answer to this is because I know assessments have to be done in the early stages, but it is the early stages when it is most difficult to establish a relationship, and being passed on and on doesn't encourage a therapeutic relationship.

The next leap of faith was going to see the analyst. When I first met her she explained she was doing an assessment of me and then I would go on a waiting list for treatment. She got full marks for that explanation, which I understood fully. But again that meant I couldn't make the leap of faith. I didn't think, 'This is it'. Instead, I thought I'd have to try and keep the lid on it all, because I would be out on my own again soon. It was many weeks before I asked how long the assessment period would take, as this cut-off point – which I thought was imminent – was experienced as a threatening presence. Only then did the analyst tell me that I was 'in therapy'. She had decided I couldn't wait. With hindsight I'm sure she was right, but I wish she'd told me earlier of her decision. All along I needed reassurance of what was expected of me, and what I could expect from the therapist.

A leap in the dark?

By inviting you to trust me I was, in a sense, inviting you to believe in me. However, that belief in me was intended only to serve as a bridge to your own natural wisdom; the wisdom of self-belief. However, stepping out onto that bridge was a significant step, given all that had gone before, and involved a clear leap of faith.

It is a truism that trusting others, no matter how difficult, is often easier than trusting ourselves. We know what is involved in trusting others. They represent something 'out there', to relate to. Relating to ourselves is more complex, perhaps because of the abstract reality of 'who' we are.

In therapy, the assumption is that the client (or patient) is lost and the therapist somehow knows the road home. Although the notion of people 'finding themselves' in therapy now has a distinctly '60s ring to it, I still believe that self-discovery is the ultimate endpoint of therapy. However, different people (and therapists) have different ideas as to what form that discovery might take. Still, reaching an understanding of a problem and how to live with it, or perhaps transcend it, involves accessing the Buddha's notion of the 'lamp within'. Carl Rogers offered an elegant modern version of the Buddha's concept when he wrote (Kirschenbaum and Henderson, 1990):

> All individuals have within themselves the ability to guide their own lives
> in a manner that is both personally satisfying and socially constructive. In
> a particular type of helping relationship, we free the individuals to find their
> inner wisdom and confidence, and they will make increasingly healthier
> and more constructive choices.

Rogers was followed by a whole range of humanistic therapists, all of whom espoused what was seen as 'unrealistic assumptions' about the nature of Man within the Freudian canon. Freud had believed to the very end of his life that humankind was fundamentally bad. The therapies that issued from Freudian thinking provided a secular version of St Augustine's belief in 'original sin'. The humanistic therapies would have no truck with this humanely pessimistic outlook, but chose instead to believe that people had the capacity to heal themselves. However, they recognized that some help was invariably needed with this project. Rogers believed that people needed someone else to accept the client's 'awful feelings'. Once this had been achieved, then they might be accepted by the client her or himself.

Although many therapists, from different 'schools' of therapy, claim to employ 'Rogerian' principles in their work, the theoretical basis of the therapy often appears to restrict their practice of the kind of trust of the patient that Rogers talked of. You had some experience of this with the analyst.

My big leap of faith with the analyst was on what turned out to be the last day I saw her. She stopped seeing me for three months when I told her I was going on holiday to Australia, although I was only going for three weeks. I assumed I had cocked up her treatment plan by taking this vacation. Anyway, for the three months I didn't get to see her I reassured myself with the knowledge that she had made an appointment to see me a week after I came back off holiday.

When I was flying back, I had what for me was a really nasty experience. The man sitting next to me kept pushing his body against mine and mauling me. It was very distressing. Eventually I passed out cold – literally! It was my period, but I think it was sheer terror that led me to pass out. Anyway, when I went to see the analyst right after that, I decided I really wanted to make the treatment work and I knew it was my fault it hadn't worked thus far because I couldn't talk. So I decided before I ever went in, I would talk and I would make it work. I took a giant leap of faith. At the time, the leap I was taking seemed like the second kind (trusting her), but in truth it was the first kind again – desperation. I told her in detail what happened on the plane and how it was such a big deal to me. I really felt like we were finally getting somewhere. I did feel better for just having talked about it. That was, until she told me not to come again until I had something I was prepared to talk about. I was devastated, and felt terribly isolated and abandoned. This sense of rejection was a serious problem for me, and I had experienced this previously with the counsellor. When the patient spills something very important and the therapist gives the impression it's not good enough, it feels like rejection or abandonment. It's like the therapist decides what's serious, what's distressing. It's just 'denial' on my part if I disagree. That's a real no-win situation.

I still feel cheated over that truly major revelation. When I came to you a few days later, how I ever got up the courage to make a leap of faith after that I'll never know, but I did. That was a 'back to the wall' type of leap. I definitely felt like I was teetering over the abyss and you were the only one around. At the time, I had no way of knowing you had a lifebelt.

There is a stereotype of the Rogerian therapeutic stance that oozes sweetness and light, with the therapist (or more often a counsellor) blandly reflecting back every word uttered by the patient or client. This caricature of Rogers' method is not only laughable, but also unworkable. It doesn't lead anywhere, and both client and therapist find themselves at a point of no return, pretty fast. If Rogers illustrated one key feature of the therapeutic relationship, it was how 'being there' for the client could be turned into an effective sounding board for the client's own thoughts and feelings. By being accessible, aiming to communicate understanding through empathy, and by being warm, without taking over the person's experience, the client often begins to feel a new-found degree of security. By accepting the person without judgement, the therapist hopes that the person will come to accept herself as a reflection of that process.

These ways of 'being with' someone in distress – even when the distress is controlled or concealed – engenders a degree of trust that eventually loops back into the client as a means of developing self-trust.

Early on in therapy you confessed how the development of the relationship with me was still tied up with other 'unfinished business' from your work with the analyst.

Friday, July 3 10.30 pm

Dear Dr B,

What a difference half an hour makes! When you saw me leaving work today I had just about thrown in the towel.

Things started to go badly wrong during a trip to my GP on Wednesday. To start off with, the GP I have been dealing with this last year was on holiday. I got a woman doctor, but someone I did not know. She had to pore over my file and quiz me a bit to get the picture. That was bad enough, but what really screwed me up were the readings taken from the analyst's letter to the GP after my last session.

The GP has concluded that Dr A and I have a communication problem. After my trip to the surgery, I would say that is a massive understatement. The problem is, we don't seem to communicate at all. We don't even seem to speak the same language!

The only reason I went to the GP was because I thought I was finished with the analyst and I wanted to come off her drugs. She (the analyst) told me I would have to go to the GP to get them reduced gradually, and that she would write to the GP about this.

I strolled into the surgery expecting it all to be sorted out and that I would get some quick instructions and a new, reduced prescription. Instead, this unfamiliar GP was not keen to vary the prescription. Dr A had said NOTHING about it in her letter.

But what the analyst did say was that she thinks I need the support of nursing staff in the setting of the day hospital or on an inpatient basis. She told the GP I have refused such treatment. The bit about inpatient care and treatment is a bombshell. She had never mentioned this to me. That, I definitely would not have forgotten about, and you certainly would have heard about it before now. As for refusing the day hospital, I had tried to explain to her more than once that I wasn't refusing the option, I just wanted information on what went on there and with whom before I made a decision on whether to get involved. My concern was mostly about having to start again with a different doctor. It seems to me I get so far and no further so many times. I wasn't prepared to let myself in for more of the same. All I wanted from the analyst was more information, and I don't think that was an unreasonable request. Nevertheless,

it was not forthcoming, and she chose to believe I was refusing her rec-
ommendations. Yes, I am angry with her for that. I was trying to be
straight with her, but she wasn't playing fair with me.

Anyway the result of all that was the GP told me to keep going with the
drugs and go back in two weeks 'once you've decided what to do'. It was
like I had to go back to the GP and say whether I was going to go to the
day hospital or get myself committed. She did say to talk it over with you
first, though, as the analyst and I obviously had a communication
problem.

Until lunchtime today I couldn't think of anything else. I had actually
decided to put my affairs in order and just go into hospital for a couple
of weeks. Incredibly, it seemed the easiest way out at the time. With
hardly any sleep since Tuesday night, and the thought of all this buzzing
around in my head, I just wanted to give up the fight and give in to a psy-
chiatric bed.

Also, all the small progresses I was so pleased about in my last letter
seemed to evaporate. I couldn't remember anything. I was making silly
mistakes, and I couldn't concentrate on a book or my work. To be honest,
I don't think there was enough space left in my head. It was all taken over
by the idea of a hospital bed.

Anyway, I went AWOL from work at lunchtime today and ended up at
home, where I found the letter from you, which had just arrived. It was
like getting an exercise back with a gold star from the teacher! I went to
the top of the class and felt heaps better. Your letter was so encouraging.
Not only did you understand what I was trying to say, but also you actu-
ally seemed to appreciate the way I was communicating. You'll never
know how much that lifted me.

One of the challenges for me in therapy is to work out how to make that
connection – how to meet the person exactly where she is, rather than
where I would like her to be. Good old-fashioned Chinese pragmatism
seems justified – if something doesn't work do something else, do anything else, but don't go over stony ground again and again. Traditional
psychiatric practice has a lot of stoical elements embedded within it. If
medication doesn't work, we often give more of the same. If therapy once
a week doesn't appear to deliver, we offer it twice a week. Sometimes this
striving to be helpful ends up being counterproductive.

One of the great mavericks of psychotherapy, Milton Erickson, largely
threw away the psychotherapeutic rulebook and dived in to where he
thought the patient actually was. It would appear that most times he dived
in at a crucial spot (O'Hanlon and Hexum, 1990). Of course, diving in
frightens many therapists, and I not infrequently simply dip my toe in. I
hope that I am dipping my toe into the same part of the pool in which the
client is swimming – or drowning. Standing hollering from the bank or
shore isn't much use, and although the client may not know *why* this is
useless, invariably she can feel the truth of her senses. It would appear

that you felt that truth, and felt somehow disempowered (to use a popular buzzword) as a result.

My letter, saying what I thought of our session and offering some encouragement for your work 'out there' in the world that led you to therapy, was a pretty straightforward affair. Maybe sending encouraging letters is so straightforward it looks crooked compared to traditional therapeutic practice. I guess I had come to the conclusion that words were important to you, and were maybe even more meaningful when they were written down.

When I told my friend Helen that I had written to you and I felt better for it, she was very wary. She thought it was a bad idea, and warned me that that was a trap I got into with the counsellor. She never approved of him, and thought he was just fleecing me for a lot of money I couldn't afford. Now I am beginning to come round to her way of thinking.

Anyway, I used to write to the counsellor a lot because I know I am much more articulate via the written rather than the spoken word. In fact, I often quite literally dry up when I am trying to say difficult things. I lose all saliva in my mouth, and I just can't make the words come out. Also I find it is often the case that I don't always fully appreciate points in a session, but I will come home, chew things over and then want to continue, but I am on my own. Writing is like picking up the conversation again and amplifying some points. The counsellor always had difficulty with this, primarily because he was dyslexic, but also I think because letters were 'stolen' time, not dealt with and paid for in the contracted hour. He also saw writing as a cop-out, and didn't really value what couldn't be spoken. This was frustrating for me because, as you seem to appreciate, some of my hardest (in my book, most valuable) work was done in the letters. To add insult to injury, he would not take his cue for a following session from a letter. He kept banging on about the 'non directive approach'. All that means to me is that I have to do all the work. What was he getting paid for?

One of the things I'm fairly certain about is that therapy is invariably a case of 'horses for courses'[1]. Your bad experiences with the counsellor and the analyst showed that these approaches were not meeting your needs, perhaps because these approaches were not connecting with you in the way that you wanted or needed. Perhaps the counsellor's 'abandonment' was a belated realization that his 'non-directive' approach was simply not for you. The analyst seemed to come to a similar conclusion, although you never did get as clear a message from her.

---

[1]Increasingly, arguments are made in favour of 'this' and against 'that' kind of therapy, often on the basis of how long it takes to effect some highly specific change. Many of these arguments claim to be about science, but I can't help feeling that they are about good old-fashioned power; the power involved in being 'right'.

Without making a conscious decision, I opted for something completely different. My therapeutic philosophy is fairly simple – like Erickson and Rogers, I believe that therapy should aim to liberate the client's potential for self-help. The focus needs to be on recognizing the uniqueness of the person, emphasizing the need to offer an original therapeutic response, rather than slavishly following some doctrinaire, orthodox methodology. In short, if something works, do more of it. If it doesn't, do something else, as I noted above. Something in your manner, rather than in your story, suggested the idea of coach–athlete. The critical reader might say that I used this analogy to play down my power over you. Perhaps! But if this was the case, that was no bad thing. Patients are sufficiently disempowered by their experiences. They don't need further limits imposed on them (however unwittingly) by therapists.

Now, I think some of the problem with the analyst is a hangover from all of that. Their approaches are too similar. I tried to discuss that with her once, but she took it as an insult. It wasn't meant to be. But you have got the point. I don't need someone to say 'Mmm'. I keep saying, if I knew what to do myself, I wouldn't be wasting a consultant's time. Now the coach/athlete approach I can accept. It's not a question of wanting to find an easy solution. Nobody would accuse Liz McColgan of being a slouch, but she benefits from a coach. All the Olympians do. The athlete has to do the hard work, but she goes to the expert, who's put people through their paces before and knows what to expect from other methods when something's not working NO MATTER HOW MUCH EFFORT THE ATHLETE'S PUTTING IN. Most of all, the coach can step back and analyse where the problem is and make alternative suggestions for a MORE APPROPRIATE training method.

Now, far from being despondent, your letter has set me back on the track with my second wind. Now I really think I can win again. A lot of that is just having confidence in yourself and your trainer and, as you said, if you've done the warm-up properly, you'll be fit for the race.

When I was going to see the analyst, I would come out hardly able to stand up sometimes. I dreaded going, dreaded what was going to happen in the sessions. Mind you, it was never as bad as I imagined it would be. Helen said I would get to the stage where I would look forward to going. I never did, but it's true when I come to see you. Last session was very, very hard for me, but when I left, though I was very tired, I felt much lighter and quite happy to walk out into a concourse full of people. I do look forward to getting back into 'hard training' with you. I know if I don't get it right first time, you have the patience and imagination to adapt the lesson to suit me.

My friend works with people who have speech problems, and she told me the best communicators are people who don't keep repeating exactly what the receiver is misunderstanding. The best communicators will find a different way to say the same thing, avoiding the words that are obvi-

ously not being picked up. I think a good therapist/coach must operate in the same way. The counsellor used to tell me I spoke a foreign language and that I persistently misunderstood him. This was very demoralizing when I was trying really hard. Maybe I shouldn't have taken all the blame and accepted it was me who was stupid and suffering from a psychotic illness. Maybe he just wasn't adaptive enough to use what I was giving him.

One of the best bits in your letter was the bit about using my mountain image to explain therapy to your other patients. I have had a hard time accepting so much help. The reason I went private initially was because I know there are loads of people with far worse problems than me who have to manage on their own because there aren't enough NHS therapists. Also, I didn't want the fact I was receiving psychiatric treatment to go on record. How can I justify taking up time when there are concentration camp survivors who need your help? Also, I know I am painfully slow. But today I have come to think of therapy with you as a privilege I can get a lot out of, and I should try to squeeze as much out of it as I can. From what you said, it won't be totally selfish if I have some talent that can be used to project the lessons more readily to other ordinary patients like me. I would feel much more at ease with therapy if I thought I was giving you something, and not just taking.

We are already into tomorrow now; 12.55 am. Now I have got this all off my chest I am proposing to do some real relaxing and forget about the homework meantime. This past week has taken a lot out of me; I haven't been eating well and certainly haven't been sleeping well. I don't have to go back to work until Tuesday afternoon. When this letter is finished I intend to sleep as long as I need to, even if that is until tomorrow afternoon. I think a weekend of snoozing and trash videos might be just what's needed before moving on to the next phase of intense training.

Sorry to take up so much of your time reading my screeds, but it saves me from feeling I need an appointment urgently. If I couldn't have written to you, it would've been a disaster that you had to cancel (the appointment). Now I can see you when I see you.

Keep on being different. I can really relate to that!

Bobbie

Early in my career I used to hope that patients would think that I looked as if I knew what I was doing, or what was happening for them, and that this appearance would instil enough confidence for them to 'take the leap'. In time I became more sophisticated with this presentation of my therapeutic self, and so gaining that trust became easier. When I became the 'Doctor', the status afforded by that ancient word probably reassured a few more patients. However, in time I came to the realization that if I wasn't asking myself 'why should anyone trust me?' – indeed, 'would I trust me?' – then the whole process might well go off the rails. When I became confident of my own lack of confidence, I became more comfortable with 'just being me', and therapy became more creative, collaborative and constructive – working *with* people taking those 'leaps of faith'. The parallel with Butch Cassidy and the Sundance Kid jumping into the raging torrent in the film of that name is perhaps a hackneyed and exaggerated comparison, but I think that it suggests the nature of the task.

Leaping from path to path

On one occasion I must have been giving this some particular thought, for I sent you a copy of some pages from Carlos Castenada. For many people, Castenada was something of an enigma. The lessons Castenada learned from his Yaqui spirit guide *Don Juan* might seem to many readers to be an odd kind of recommended reading for a woman reared in a Presbyterian community, who was just trying to get to grips with an emotional life that had 'gone off the rails'. However, this was just one example of a 'leap of faith' on my part, hoping that you would find Castenada's reflections apposite (Castenda, 1968):

> All paths are the same: they lead nowhere. They are all paths going through the bush, or into the bush. In my own life I could say I have traversed long, long paths. But I am not anywhere. My benefactor's question has meaning now. Does this path have a heart? If it does, the path is good: if it doesn't it is of no use. Both paths lead nowhere; but one has a heart, the other doesn't. One makes for a joyful journey; as long as you follow it, you are one with it. The other will make a curse of your life. One makes you strong; the other weakens you. ... For me there is only the travelling on paths that have heart, on any path that may have heart. There I travel, and the only worthwhile challenge is to traverse its full length. And there I travel, looking, looking, breathlessly.

One of the risks I expected you to take involved exposing yourself to powerful emotions. For me, the path with heart had always meant the path that led back home. It appeared to go 'out' somewhere into the world, but really only looped back on itself, taking you to within sight of the 'lamp within'. It was also appropriate to acknowledge that I was inviting you to engage in rigorous discipline. In one letter, I drew a discrete parallel between the hard work of sports training[2] and therapy:

> ... I was also interested in the way that you recognized some of the changes that have occurred over the months ... Noticing these changes is, in a sense,

---

[2] I chose the sporting analogy with its related metaphors, since I knew that you enjoyed sports.

akin to recognizing that you are ready or prepared to do something strenu-
ous, like recognizing that you warmed up properly before running a race.
Sure you can say that you only completed the warm-up. The warm-up may,
however, be the key to success or failure in the race itself. Pooh pooh at
your own peril.

It is enormously reassuring to see evidence that you are working on your
life problems in everyday life. I recognize that the sessions, important
thought they are, symbolize the coaching metaphor. We work out some
strategies, we discuss some problems, we do a bit of 'heavy training' which
you find very taxing; then you go off and apply what you have learned in
your life game. It's not often that I work with some one who can describe
so articulately how they are doing this. Keep up the good work.

The virtue of blind faith

One morning a letter arrived in my post, which indicated quite clearly
that you had come to trust me. Indeed, you appeared to have crossed a
very significant trust barrier.

Wednesday, January 27

Dear Phil,

*We will have to agree to stop, otherwise there will be no ending. Your
ideas so excite me that I feel we could go on forever. With each contact
we seem to excite some novel trains of thought which stimulate and
sustain others when we are alone.*

*Lots of thoughts today since receiving my bumper fun pack this
morning. Thanks very much for that. When I read your letter I cried. I
can't explain why (does there have to be a reason?), and when I read it
again later in the day I didn't. It was just something that happened. It
didn't frighten me, embarrass me or make me feel I had to stop. It was
just 'interesting'. The funny thing is, I have spent some time in the past
trying to address the issue of not crying. I even thought it was some kind
of technique I ought to learn for relief. I studied a very interesting book
on the subject at the beginning of last year, but still tears were elusive.
So, like many things, it happened when I least expected it and when I
wasn't trying. Thank you for that.*

*I am becoming quite at ease with my 'uniqueness' – thanks again. I
have been busy constructing, deconstructing and reconstructing my
schemas since we last met, dipping into your book again and getting a
lot from your talk about discovering the 'joy of ordinariness'. Tonight I
felt like going out for a walk, not a run (because I couldn't face a pile of
sweaty clothes to clean afterwards), but just a walk. It was raining when
I got outside. If ever anything helped me to appreciate my uniqueness, it*

was the simple pleasure of just walking in the rain (I can tell you there were few people out discovering this joy).

Your ideas on discovery and creativity were meandering through my head while the raindrops were dancing on it. It seems to me that many people have lost the joy of ordinary creativity in our society. This weekend, I discovered the ability to create soup. Don't laugh, but I really do think we have been distanced from the ordinary man's creativity by the introduction of microwaveable pre-packed ready meals, and the throwaway philosophy that prevents a man fixing an iron or a kettle because the manufacturer has designed it in such a way that it can't be repaired but must be replaced. Many simple satisfactions are now denied us in this way.

Another simple creative pleasure I have returned to recently is knitting. Bet you didn't see me as a knitter! It is always cheaper to go out and buy a jumper for my weans[3], but never as satisfying. They think I am so clever(!) and of course it means the garment is unique, if only because of a different set of colours chosen from the pattern.

Yes, I think I am at the point of no return. I am going to be a personal scientist[4] all my days!

Had a dip into the running book too tonight. I found an echo of my ideas on not wanting to feel I HAVE TO run a certain distance, or go sub-four. You would think I'd been talking to the guy. Back to the 'there are only three original jokes' theory, eh?

Finally, before I go off and curl up with Anthony Clare's new book, I recall your words: 'Even as I write this letter I have no way of knowing what it might mean to you'. You should know that it means much, makes me feel brave and without fear, an explorer about to set out on an unknown, eagerly anticipated journey. I believe you will find that enough.

Your disciple,

Bobbie

PS A therapist once tried to tell me we were equals. It came across as learned jargon, trotted out pat. In your presence I have felt it to be true, and have learned to trust my feelings.

Perhaps I should have been pleased, since therapists devote so much time to negotiating trust. A few days later I framed some of that unease in a short letter:

---

[3]Reference to the children you looked after each week.

[4]I had talked about Michael Mahoney's notion of the 'Personal Scientist', where the patient studies her or himself in search of solutions, rather than being studied by the therapist as an object. Like many of these references to 'bright ideas', you assumed that this was one of mine. Another example, perhaps, of how therapists might acquire power and status by association.

Dear Bobbie

Many thanks for your letter. Apologies for using the word processor; I have something to say and would rather that you could read it easily.

You offer me an enormous compliment by suggesting that you might in any way be my disciple. I am the disciple of Uncertainty: she has always served me well; reminding me that each and every moment is *the* moment within which I shall have the opportunity to determine the direction of the rest of my life. I began life as a child of the Roman Catholic faith. I now no longer have any need for faith for, as Jung said, now 'I know'. But the knowledge is Uncertainty – knowing that there is nothing to know, but everything to discover. Even as I write this short letter I have no way of knowing what it might mean to you. Suffice to say that I have valued your position as my 'disciple'. I have learned much from working with you. Who knows what the future might offer. I would *hope* for friendship and camaraderie. I shall wait to see what Uncertainty brings in her heady wake.

The idea that we can turn to our inner wisdom in moments of crisis is now well accepted. Well, I should say that almost everyone repeats the Rogerian mantra, but I often wonder how many really *believe* in the way Rogers did. How many have really taken the leap of faith. Just about everywhere one looks, people are seeking new solutions to old problems – quicker ways, more effective ways, even 'scientifically validated' methods. This is certainly evident in the 'new age' scene, but is probably just as evident in the psychotherapy literature, where there is much jockeying for position in the race for the title of the perfect therapy. Some of this appears to be a function of our secular society. If there are to be no pearly gates, no eternal light at the end of life's dark tunnel, maybe we should seek some kind of 'heaven on earth' (Storm, 1991). So wherever we look we see crystal-swinging alternative lifestyles and mind-bending belief systems, all promising to improve you, enhance you, make you better, help you self-actualize, and ultimately give you heaven on earth. I have long felt that this yearning for fulfilment was little more than a sign of the emptiness of our lives from which we seek to escape. And so I settled on a simpler, more direct path to something closer to home: the lamp within.

Ralph Waldo Emerson had visited this path before – indeed, about 150 years ago. He tried to put his own spin on the Buddha's call to self-sufficiency:

Man is timid and apologetic; he is no longer upright; he dares not say 'I think', 'I am', but quotes some saint or sage[5]. He is ashamed before the blade of grass and blowing rose. These roses under my window make no reference to former roses or to better ones; they are what they are; they exist with God today. There

---

[5]The irony of my repeated citation of sages or saints is not lost on me.

is no time to them. There is simply the rose; it is perfect in every moment of its existence ... But man postpones or remembers; he does not live in the present but with reverted eye laments the past or, heedless of the riches that surround him, stands on tiptoe to foresee the future. He cannot be happy and strong until he too lives with nature in the present above time. (Emerson, 1993)

I never doubted for one moment how difficult that particular challenge might be for you: to live *in* the moment, *for* the moment. I had spent much of my adult life trying to acquire that particular 'trick of being ordinary' (Brandon, 1989). However, I had taken that leap of faith, and it was a leap from which it was impossible to return. I believed that you would find your own resolution within yourself, and would find your own path of the heart. I also believed that the way (the Tao) to that knowledge required you to grow your awareness of your self, your world, your emotional reactions and your thoughts – among other things. But first you needed to get things in perspective. This was not my judgement, but your own. You repeatedly described how everything had grown 'out of proportion' and, as a result, you knew that you had lost the vital sense of perspective.

Freud, who in this book keeps cropping up as both a hero and a villain, was aware towards the end of his life of how people were slowly but surely losing the plot. In his last great work, *Civilization and its Discontents* (quoted in Gay, 1995) he noted:

> It is impossible to escape the impression that people commonly use false standards of measurement – that they seek power, success and wealth for themselves and admire it in others, and they underestimate what is of true value in life.

Freud concluded that the only important things in life were *love* and *work*. The elusive goal of happiness was, in his view, achievable by the most old-fashioned of lifestyle tactics:

> No other technique for the conduct of life attaches the individual so firmly to reality as laying emphasis on work; for work offers a secure place in a portion of reality, in the human community ... the human relations connected with it lends a value by no means second to what it enjoys as something indispensable to the preservation and justification of existence in society.

As we worked together I gained the impression that you 'knew' what Freud had known, but that your awareness of this personal wisdom – the lamp within – was somehow just out of sight. Through focusing on awareness and the everyday business of 'noticing', I hoped that you would release the shade from that lamp within.   .

And so we set about focusing on 'noticing'. There was no expectation that you would notice anything of any great significance. Indeed, the sheer insignificance of what you would notice belied its significance – as David Kline, the Amish farmer, discovered. He described the pressures put on Amish farmers to introduce herbicides into their farms, Kline begged an all too significant question for all of us: 'Should we (the Amish) give up the kind of farming that has been proven to preserve communities and land and is ecologically and spiritually sound for a way that is culturally and environmentally harmful?' He decided that the answer was simple yet profound – No! David Kline was being tempted in much the same way that Adam had been encouraged to tempt Eve. By resisting the temptation, he kept himself open to the messages from reality that are largely lost from the existence of most of us. Speaking of the presumed drudgery of work – ploughing in particular – he wrote (Kline, 1993):

> Maybe I'm blind, but no matter which angle I look from, I fail to see any drudgery in this work. ... Several springs ago – actually it was in late winter – following a week of unseasonably warm weather, our neighbour to the south couldn't resist the urge any longer and started ploughing. I wasn't aware of it until, while walking to the barn, I suddenly caught the aroma of newly turned earth. I stood there, closed my eyes, and revelled in till, the promise of spring.

It seems unremarkable that David Kline should live a happy life. As he said:

> It was a good day. As a friend said recently, 'All days are good – some are just better than others'.

You took to the 'noticing' approach like a duck to water:

Wednesday, December 2

I've just had a 'just bathing' session. It was really good. No radio on, no distractions, just relaxing in the water 'til I was aware my feet and fingers were prunes!

Last night I spent the entire evening on the settee 'just lying' (as I had some painful menstrual cramps).

When I came home tonight, I went out 'just running'. Tried to run with long, relaxed strides from the hip and keep the shoulders loose. That was hardest. Had to keep coming back to concentrate on shoulders.

Next, I did something totally unusual for me – 'just cooking'. Made a proper meal and even had it sitting down at a table. Funny, I didn't get a lot of sleep last night because of painful cramps, but I am less knackered having had this different evening than if I had come in and just flopped in front of the TV. I feel really perky and ready to do a few more activi-

ties. Also I have decided doing ordinary things differently can give you a boost – like having a bath at teatime when it is usually part of the morning rush routine, listening to a different radio station, or switching it off altogether.

Did some 'traffic light respite' today, but missed other opportunities. I've not trained myself to second-nature level on that yet, but I'm confident I will soon.

It may seem as if I am stretching the truth a bit – you can even call me romantic – but I am sure that David Kline would describe you as reconnecting with what's important, even when it is inanimate stuff. Growing the kind of knowledge that David Kline writes about allows you to rediscover one of Einstein's less well-known laws:

> A human being is part of the whole that we call the universe, a part limited in time and space. He experiences himself, his thoughts and feelings, as something separated from the rest – a kind of optical illusion of his consciousness. This illusion is a prison for us, restricting us to our personal desires and to affection for only the few people nearest us. Our task must be to free ourselves from this prison by widening our circle of compassion to embrace all living beings and all of nature.

Few would have classed the father of the Theory of Relativity as a 'tree-hugger', but there you are – he speaks for himself. I knew you already had compassion for other beings. Your journals had described in great detail your affection for the children in your life, to whom you gave selflessly. You also held no grudges against your family, who had 'pained' you greatly in the past and could have, with your permission, continued to pain you. All that appeared necessary to complete this compassion circle was for you to accept yourself. Perhaps the biggest challenge for all of us.

A few weeks later, your experience of 'just being' appeared to open your heart to all sorts of new-found things, even a sense of equanimity in the face of sadness:

Sunday

I had a very relaxing morning at the wheel of my car. A friend of mine asked me to look after her granddaughter, and I took her to all the places I used to take her father when I babysat for him when I was still at school – that's getting old! The wee tot started to suck her thumb and look sleepy, so I bundled her in the car and turned the heating up full. It never fails to send them into the land of nod! 'Just driving' in the country roads round my home was bliss. I saw three pheasants and a fascinating children's rope swing hanging from a tree, which had an enormous bone tied to the end for a seat. It looked like a thigh-bone from a cow, and probably was.

I was just aimlessly driving round to let the wean sleep, but ended up at a junction with a signpost saying 'Siddlestone 3/4 mile'. That is where my brother was killed. Today would have been his thirtieth birthday. I didn't go, but the point is, I wasn't scared to go. I was able to think about him quite happily, and enjoy my thoughts without them intruding on the present. I think that's okay.

Blood, sweat and tears

The work involved in therapy is hard work. Sometimes it can even be difficult for the therapist – especially when he has to deal with his great desire to be a healer, and so creates for himself an unnecessary burden. But it was you who undertook the real work, both within and without the sessions. Today, there are a whole range of therapies that promise quick solutions to longstanding problems and, it should be said, some of them appear to be successful in obtaining these limited goals – of reducing distress and opening people to more possibilities in everyday living. Invariably the person on the receiving end has little or no knowledge of what exactly has happened to effect this change in their circumstances[6]. In the beginning, I don't think that you had too much idea of what was happening. You hoped that I might be of some use to you. You hoped that I might be able to somehow 'magic away' some of the more troubling experiences to which you were prone. I was fortunate that this was all you were looking for, as these more everyday forms of 'magic' are not too demanding a trick for the therapist. Sometimes the mere act of discharging all of your fears about troubling experiences to someone who you don't know, but who you think understands these phenomena better than you, is enough to weaken their effects.

However, it became clear that you had not developed these troubling experiences by anything like a random, meaningless, route. I wasn't sure, exactly, of the route by which you came by these problems, but I knew that you knew. I only needed to gain your confidence, so that you might gain your own confidence and so confront your own demons[7]. I say 'only' by way of emphasizing how straightforward, yet complex and demanding, was the gaining of that confidence.

Metaphorically, the process of therapy involves a lot of blood and sweat and, usually literally, tears. I am not sure what kind of worthy accomplishment is achieved without the expense of this common human triumvirate.

Reflecting on this theme of 'work', you wrote:

---

[6]Whether or not the therapists *actually* know what has happened may also be open to question.

[7]In the past, psychic distress was invariably attributed to demons. Now, in our new-found wisdom, we attribute out distress to equally abstract processes – like traumatic memories, or even our neuro-chemistry – which are no less demonic in their effects.

Eventually, after some time working with you. I really wanted to get better and get on with my life. Of course this was – deep down – always my objective but, since this story is a warts-and-all tale if it is to be of any use, I am ashamed to admit that there was a sticking period both with the analyst and the counsellor. At those points I was afraid to get better. Looking back from where I am now, the status quo *was terrible, but there were great chunks of time when all I wanted was to maintain the status quo. I felt I needed the therapeutic relationship as it was, and couldn't take the risk of change. At that point I couldn't handle any 'leaps of faith'. The trouble is that with any relationship that you don't allow to change and grow, you ultimately kill it off. In a simple friendship, you can't say, 'this is a good relationship, I don't want to lose it. I'll freeze-frame it and keep it forever'. It took me a long time to learn that's the quickest way to strangle a relationship.*

I suppose what I'm saying is that therapy should always encourage a vision of the future, a vision of the independent person meeting the world with enthusiasm and confidence, ready to change and be changed.

In the beginning of therapy I was definitely looking for a 'cure' for largely unnamed ills. Now I think that it is appropriate only to seek 'healing' from the therapeutic relationship. I think that if you don't operate some kind of continuing care and maintenance programme for yourself (if you don't work at it), then there is always the risk of becoming mentally unwell again. In mind terms I will make sure that I get plenty of nourishment and exercise, truly 'fit for life'.

Fear of further failure

Of course, during therapy you became aware of all sorts of things – including things you saw as your weaknesses, your human foibles. When you are involved in a reclamation project, it can be hard and dirty work. Retrieving something of worth from among apparent rubbish is demanding and often frustrating. Some people who have been in extreme states of mental distress believe that the process of recovering one's sanity becomes a way of life. It seems true also of the more everyday business of reclaiming bits of ourselves that have been stolen or damaged in the hurly-burly of life. Pat Deegan described this recovery process elegantly (Deegan, 1988, 1993):

> Recovery does not refer to an end product or result. It does not mean that ... I (was) cured. In fact, our recovery is marked by an ever-deepening acceptance of our limitations. But now, rather than being an occasion for despair, we find that our personal limitations are the ground from which spring our own unique possibilities. This is the paradox of recovery, i.e. that in accepting what we cannot do or be, we begin to discover who we can be and what we can do. For many of us who are disabled,

recovery is a process, a way of life, an attitude, and a way of approaching the day as a challenge.

Cul de sacs

The idea of *waiting* for the resolution of a problem, far less waiting on enlightenment, is not part of our contemporary mind set. We assume that everything needs to be pursued, chased vigorously and ultimately captured. Life and the everyday business of living it has become a project; something that we do in pursuit of something else, not something we do for its own sake. Problem solving is the outstanding characteristic of human beings. We assume that problems will not resolve themselves, but will only yield to the exercise of our greater intelligence. Sometimes this is undoubtedly the case. However, by overgeneralizing we have lost our appreciation for dealing with problems by simply letting them go; waiting for them to take flight from our lives. To do nothing is the greatest challenge of all. Rilke knew the nature of this challenge (quoted in Mitchell, 1991):

> Being an artist means: not numbering and counting, but ripening like a tree, which doesn't force its sap, and stands confidently in the storms of spring, not afraid that afterward summer may not come. It does come. But it comes only to those who are patient, who are there as if eternity lay before them, so unconcernedly silent and vast. I learn it every day of my life, learn it with pain I am grateful for: *patience* is everything.

The term 'patient' has become outmoded in health care, perhaps because it denotes an unwelcome passivity. However, it seems clear that you *had* to be a 'patient' to rediscover your own person-hood through your patient-hood. The process of therapy for you was, without doubt, replete with the lessons, painfully learned, of which Rilke spoke.

Uncertainty principle revisited

The second part of the letter that began this chapter continued the theme of uncertainty. You had been writing of your 'struggle' to learn the guitar, but had also alluded to some changes in your approach to life in general, which was less focused on achieving direct goals, on producing what increasingly we call – especially in health care – 'discrete outcomes'.

> ... I feel that my work is truly finished with you when you say that 'I have no rigid plans, no point in that'. In place of rigidity you offer 'fancies' for this or that. If more people were willing to 'take a fancy to this or that', we might have less repetition, less conflict, more discovery and creativity.

Soon you will come to *discover* the guitar: so far you appear to be trying to control it, to make it *do* things *for* you. I offer you a little wisdom from one of my generation's great voices who is, fortunately, not stilled – Robert M Pirsig (Prisig, 1974):

When one isn't dominated by feelings of separateness from what he's working on, then one can be said to 'care' about what he's doing. That is what caring really is, a feeling of identification with what one's doing. When one has this feeling then he also sees the inverse side of caring, Quality itself.

And more importantly, he commented:

I think that when this concept of peace of mind is introduced and made central to the act of technical work, a fusion of classic and romantic quality can take place at a basic level within the practical working context. I've said that you can actually see this fusion in skilled mechanics and machinists of a certain sort, and you can see it in the work they do. To say that they are not artists is to misunderstand the nature of art. They have patience, care and attentiveness to what they're doing, but more than this – there's a kind of inner peace of mind that isn't contrived but results from a kind of inner harmony with the work in which there's no leader and no follower. The material and the craftsman's thoughts change together in a progression of smooth, even changes until his mind is at rest at the exact instant the material is right.

When you *let* yourself 'harmonize' with the guitar, you will discover what you learned at the 'led lite lespite'[8]: that *you* and the *guitar* cease to exist and are replaced by 'music'. Rock on!!

I closed my short epistle with a brief recognition that, despite my protestations, discipleship was not a bad thing, since I saw myself similarly as a disciple.

... I also enclose a copy of my interview with Hilda Peplau, one of the wisest people I have ever met; the other is Annie Altschul, my mentor from Edinburgh. Their wisdom is conveyed through 'comfort'. One could sleep in their presence and still be gifted with something.

I never appreciated at the time the cross-cultural significance of the reference to 'comfort' until I went to New Zealand a couple of years later.

---

[8]This was another reference to wee Malcie. You had been using the stationary period at traffic lights as a 'quiet zone', where you could relax and 'be in the moment'. And so your self-instruction – 'red light – respite!' became 'led lite, lespite'. With the irony only children are capable of, he knew what to call it but did not know what *it* was. Wittgenstein might even have laughed.

One day a white woman (*pakeha*) whose husband was Maori was driving me back to my hotel after a conference. I observed how attentive the audience had been, especially given the length of my session. She laughed and said that, to the Maori people there and people like her who had joined Maori culture, my talk was very short. The previous weekend she had been to a feast where the speeches could last up to twelve hours. How could anyone concentrate for that length of time, I asked? Her response surprised me at first, but in time I realized that intuitively I had 'known' the Maori principle:

> Oh, no-one needs to listen actively to the whole speech. People bring blankets and cushions and lie down on the floor. Some rest, others just go to sleep. Even when the audience is asleep, the Maori speaker believes that the speech is being heard.

She offered me a fine illustration of the importance of 'comfort' for listening and learning. Perhaps we too both heard what each other said and embraced it in our hearts, even if we were not necessarily 'actively listening' at the time.

A sense of personal agency

If I had to plump for one idea that somehow draws together the various outcomes of these various 'leaps of faith', it would be your acquisition of a sense of personal agency. Your various leaps into the beyond, especially when you feared what you might land on, helped you regain your own sense of personal power. There is a lot of talk today about mental health professionals 'empowering' people, but in truth all we can do is stop taking your power away from you by fostering dependence or covertly controlling you. The story-ing process, which we discussed in Chapter 2, also illustrates how, by telling and retelling your story, you took back some of that lost power by making the story *your* story once again, rather than a medicalized or psychological account of your story. In a sense, by taking charge of your story, framed in your words and phrases, you reclaimed your experience, the territory of your own distress. Through taking all of that back, you changed your whole attitude towards the 'it' that had for so long tormented you.

An Australian friend of mine has written evocatively about a similar leap of faith, which he took in relation to what often is seen as a kind of 'terminal' mental illness: schizophrenia. Simon Champ wrote:

> I began to see that while I might not be able to control my illness, I could control my attitude towards it. I began to see strong links between quality of life and the attitude one had towards illness. I became increasingly concerned with the language and attitudes expressed by many members of the

organization I had helped to start. The constant reference to people who experience schizophrenia as 'sufferers' or 'victims' of illness seemed offensive to me. While I was the first to admit that schizophrenia had dominated my life for many years and that it could indeed be a terrible disease, I also knew that I had only made progress with my recovery when I stopped seeing myself as a 'victim' and relinquished more passive roles in my treatment. 'Sufferer' was the language of victims and lacked dignity. Illness was becoming one aspect of the whole me, not the centre of me. By changing the focus of the illness in my life, I think my management of the illness was strengthened. I was indeed a person who happened to experience psychotic episodes, but I refused to be described as a 'sufferer'. Even for those of us facing great psychiatric disabilities, our souls can flower with hope.

Simon's comments about dignity seem very close to the nub of the issue. All forms of mental distress serve to alienate people from what we might call their true selves. It certainly seemed that way for you. To reclaim that lost territory requires a courageous 'leap of faith'. The reward may, however, be the re-acquisition of your sense of dignity. When you are redignified (so to speak), you can exercise again your own voice, make your own choices, do your own thing – including making your own mistakes. None of this seems to me to be about 'becoming perfect'. Indeed, one view of the concept of 'self-actualization' first framed by Maslow is not that one should become perfect, but that one should grow into the kind of person who is open to the possibilities of contact – with the whole world – that Einstein talked about. Usually that involves becoming independent of the good opinion of others – being able to live one's own life, detached from outcomes – doing things just for the sake of doing them, and having no investment in power, or control over other people. There is less and less faith in this concept in today's world, where fitting in, being focused on production and a thousand versions of the old power game are the unwritten rules of Western society. That may explain why there is so much distress in the world, and why, despite our sophisticated psychology, the rate of that distress grows with each passing day. You know there is no going back, but the way forward may, paradoxically, involve not going anywhere. The journey of a thousand miles does start under your very feet and, having leapt the 'leap of faith', maybe you found that you are back where you started. However, as Simon Champ discovered, by going nowhere perhaps you also discovered that everything changed.

References

Barker, P. (1999). *Talking Cures: A Guide to the Psychotherapies for Health Care Professionals*. NT Books.
Brandon, D. (1989). *The Trick of being Ordinary*. Mind.

Castenda, C. (1968). *The Teachings of Don Juan: A Yaqui Way of Knowledge.* Penguin.

Deegan, P. E. (1988). Recovery: the lived experience of rehabilitation. *Psychosocial Rehab. J.,* **11,** 11–19.

Deegan, P. E. (1993). Recovering our sense of value after being labelled. *J. Psychosocial Nurs. Mental Health Serv.,* **31,** 7–11.

Emerson, Ralph Waldo (1993). *Self Reliance and other Essays,* (Dover Thrift edition). Dover Publications.

Gay, P. (ed.) (1995). *The Freud Reader,* pp. 722–71. Vintage.

Kirschenbaum, H. and Henderson, V. L. (eds) (1990). *The Carl Rogers Reader,* p. xiv. Constable.

Kline, D. (1993). *Great Possessions: An Amish Farmer's Journal,* p. xix. The Sumach Press.

Mitchell, S. (1991). *The Enlightened Mind,* pp. 186–7, HarperCollins.

O'Hanlon, W. H. and Hexum, A. L. (1990). *An Uncommon Casebook: The Complete Clinical Work of Milton H. Erickson, MD.* W. W. Norton.

Pirsig, R. M. (1974). *Zen and the Art of Motorcycle Maintenance.* Corgi Books.

Storm, R. (1991). *In Search of Heaven on Earth.* Bloomsbury.

8

The glory of discovery

Drawing lessons

Drawing a parallel between therapy and education is appropriate, if a little obvious. The educator is intent not so much on teaching something, but on helping arrange the conditions under which the person might learn something of some note, something of value – probably of personal value. Such a significant kind of learning can only come from within – or at least will involve a subtle, perhaps less than obvious, restructuring and redefinition of that which already lies 'within'. You might call that the 'felt knowledge' of the person. This definition of education betrays its emphasis on *educere* – the drawing out from within. In such an education, the person metaphorically dips inside, drawing out something from the font of their own personal knowledge, bringing it into contact with the illumination possible *in the world:* the illumination that is possible only through direct experience.

I have long believed that this meaning is central to the therapeutic endeavour, for it is the person who is *to be healed*, metaphorically or perhaps even literally. You may well say that this too is obvious, but many therapeutic conversations are distorted by the failure of the therapist to appreciate this simple fact – a failing that is compounded by notions of the healing 'power' of the therapist. Ever since Freud made his alleged 'discoveries' about the nature and the functions of the unconscious, therapists have often been sorely tempted to 'fix' the patient[1]. The brief is more important than this, yet simpler: to provide the condi-

---

[1] The way that therapists 'restate' people's experiences – attempting to give something with its inherent meaning some other kind of meaning, a socially-validated or normalized meaning – was part of Foucault's critique of the psychiatric institution. Psychotherapy, like its godfather psychiatry, risks promulgating the view that there *is* one single truth concerning the human condition, whereas in everyday fact people construct their own meanings in the course of their life narrative.

tions under which the patient might be healed by Nature or by God[2]. Therapy can entail, therefore, a search to establish what is important for the patient, not for the therapist. Regrettably, therapists risk working on themselves and their own needs rather than those of the person who is the patient. In addition to ensuring that the person is given a good 'hearing', the therapist needs to listen intently for signs of discovery – invariably signalled by the events surrounding whatever happens when the penny drops.

When true education happens, the experience may signal itself – but rarely in the direct, concrete way signalled by the experience of successful training. The person who experiences an educational *happening* comes to 'know' something; becomes something of a personal epistemologist. She moves from holding opinions about herself and her experience to 'just knowing' that what she believes is indeed true. She might call the acquisition of such a personal wisdom an 'ah-hah experience', but it is likely to be less flashy, sudden or startling in its illumination. More likely, it just dawns on her that this (now) is the case, and from then on there is no turning back.

Thursday, 7.30 pm

It's about time I brought all the rush of ideas, enthusiasm and theories under some sort of control, brought discipline to bear. Help the patient heal herself. The thing I am noticing at the moment is a feeling of bigness. If 'bigness' isn't in the dictionary, then I've invented it. It means a feeling of bursting with plans, jumping from one project to the next, and of success breeding success. I don't necessarily mean big success, but little successes give a feeling of bigness; a feeling that there's more to come, an expectant feeling, a joyous anticipation.

Many of the little successes that have happened recently haven't been specifically anticipated, and what I'm noticing at the moment is the need to be open to new experience. As a friend of mine used to say, 'Just go with the flow'. I think that in the past that has always been an almost negative attitude, and therefore not acceptable to me, but now I choose to interpret it as meaning, don't be too rigid. Leave yourself open to unexpected challenges and experiences, and enjoy the bigness of being absorbed into new and unexpected areas of development.

I was just sitting in the bath half an hour ago, thinking what a good time I'm having at the moment, and a couple of ideas came into my head for work. I thought to myself, 'This isn't my usual kind of stuff', and then I decided, 'Give it a go. It might become your kind of stuff'. I'm really aware of a feeling of not wanting to be limited at the moment, to keep the elasticity in my boundaries, and keep poking out in new bounces.

---

[2]I am reminded that this form of words is not far from the original lines of Florence Nightingale when she talked of what could be accomplished by nursing.

But being realistic, I have to allow the other side of this – fear of failure. At the moment, because I'm up, it's just a wee harmless fly, but to pretend it's not there is to let it grow into a great big, horrible, hairy spider some day. In a way we spoke about just this thing quite early on in our knowing each other. I remember you putting a coin up on the desk and saying that the tension of two seemingly mutually exclusive ideas, which I was experiencing, was just the two faces of the same coin – happy and sad, that sort of thing.

I have been experiencing little hits of fear of failure about work. I think that is because when ideas are bursting out and working out, it points up the contrast when you're short on ideas, bored, frustrated. These feelings also feed on themselves, and I am scared of getting into a downward spiral.

I hear you drawing out (from within) some old, pretty well-worn characterizations of yourself. It sounds almost as if you have drawn them out and held them up to the light – the light being this new-found 'bigness'. Your joy – experienced in the bigness – is that these older characterizations of yourself seem to have lost much of their power in the light of your new-found 'bigness'.

But the joy of such bigness also has its down side, as you realize that your buoyancy might only heighten your sensitivity to any negative strike – and negative strikes (in your version of the world) are *bound* to come some day; likely some day soon. I have long wondered about this way of representing reality, not least because I have done it myself, over and over again down the years. How can we *know* that there will be 'negative strikes'? I guess you might say, 'because they have happened in the past'. That's the old probabilistic version of the world – history has a habit of repeating itself. But how do we know this to be true? If we did not know our own history, would it repeat itself? Well, obviously not, because we wouldn't see events as a repetition, only as an 'event' – as a happening. And of course, happenings are things that we might learn from (*educere*).

The American Morita therapist, David Reynolds, was asked if he had found enlightenment by studying the ways of his Japanese masters. He replied: 'Sometimes I'm like this and sometimes I'm like that' (Reynolds, 1987). Some might read this as avoidance, but it reads like genuine wisdom to me. Reynolds draws on his experience, recognizing that life has no hidden meanings, but only the significance that *we* attach to life and our living of it. The drawing lesson that Reynolds has clearly learned is that Reality is the master and he, as the student, must take every opportunity that Reality offers to learn what 'needs to be done'. And of course, he learns that 'sometimes he is like this, and (at other times) is like that'.

Our scientifically minded society harbours a vain belief that reality can somehow be changed, adapted or manipulated. However, the reality of Reality is somewhat simpler and more profound. Western thought has taught us that the first step in controlling something is to understand it, then to act on this knowledge (theory) to make it change. As Reynolds notes (Reynolds, 1985):

> Of course we run into all sorts of difficulties with this approach whenever we encounter something that cannot be understood rationally – death, for example, and emotions (such as love and despair) and the sacred. We aren't taught the usefulness of accepting reality, both that part of it that we can change and that part that we can't. We may see acceptance as a sort of giving up, a last resort. In fact, acceptance of the way things are is always the first step in changing things. Denial of reality, resistance to reality, fantasies, and even elaborate plans don't accomplish change.

I have used the metaphor 'drawing' several times during my reflections. It is a fine word, rather like a pencil, having so many diverse uses. However, as I reflect I sense that what I am picking up in your reflections on your experiences is more than metaphor. There does appear to be a drawing lesson taking place, but what is the subject – if not the object – of your lesson?

To answer my own question, I turn to some drawings that Leonardo executed towards the end of his life, or so it is commonly thought. They are commonly called the 'deluge' drawings, suggesting an association with the biblical flood, but probably Leonardo was simply intrigued with the torrential energy of what we might call 'a good downpour'. Because these drawings contain some tiny figures and even horses apparently being tossed in Leonardo's tautly drawn maelstrom, many have interpreted these as an apocalyptic vision of the world's end. Leonardo's notebooks[3], however, suggest an altogether more empirical vision, though no less full of awe and foreboding. The drawings seem to illustrate how Leonardo, even in the twilight of his life, continued to study and marvel at the power of nature. Observation of the rules of nature were a long-standing preoccupation of his notebooks, recognizing repeatedly the power of water to shape mountains and, ultimately, to prove their undoing. Leonardo appreciated that men might control water to a degree, but ultimately it had the power to overwhelm any human enterprise. Things are no different today, despite 500 years of subsequent human achievement.

Perhaps Leonardo sat down to execute those sixteen drawings as a kind of meditation on what he saw as the ultimate power of the nature he had assiduously studied for most of his life. His meditation led him to a conclusion not far from the modern day serenity prayer, which extemporized on the opportunity for control of our destiny, within the context of acceptance of our fate. Perhaps Machiavelli's *Prince* was one of the first to flesh out the drawing lesson that Leonardo was taking (Machiavelli, 1961):

---

[3] I am indebted to Richard Turner's analysis for my perspective on the deluge drawings (Turner, 1993).

Nonethless, so as not to rule out our free will, I believe that it is probably true that fortune is the arbiter of half the things we do, leaving the other half or so to be controlled by ourselves. I compare fortune to one of those violent rivers which, when they are enraged, flood the plains, tear down trees and buildings, wash soil from one place to deposit it in another. Everyone flees before them, everybody yields to their impetus, there is no possibility of resistance. Yet although such is their nature, it does not follow that when they are flowing quietly one cannot take precautions, constructing dykes and embankments so that when the river is in flood they would keep to one channel or their impetus would be less wild and dangerous. So it is with fortune.

And so you too, appear to be drawing much the same conclusions.

Needs, wants and wishes

August 20, 10.40 pm

Do you know I even thought at one point about going to the boss and saying we should drop a particular project because S didn't like it? It really was a temptation, because it would be an 'acceptable' way to fail. It would relieve me of the weekly agony of starting with a blank page and wanting desperately to reach a high standard. But it would also relieve me of the joy of being told I've done something good, and it would limit me by shrinking me back to what I knew was achievable and not enlarging into what might *be achievable.*

Now is possibly the time to admit I have 'a record of previous convictions' for taking the easy way out. When I was at university, I wasn't really a good student. Though I need time on my own every day, I am basically a people person and thrive on the stimulus of working with others. With only five hours a week of scheduled lectures and tutorials, I was dying of loneliness at Uni. Sitting in a library with a few hundred people can be a very lonely experience. Despite all the people around you, you have only your own thoughts to think. When my sister died, I got out. I knew people would say it was because of her. I wasn't being a 'real' dropout. Like I say, I can kid myself there is an 'acceptable' way to fail. I suppose I've been aware of this for years, but I'm still not making any effort to square the circle. Can you reflect that back to me in any helpful way?

Sorry I am going on so much. Hope it is not too much for you, but I am finding it helpful to work via this book. It's probably not the homework that was set, but I hope you can bear with me. Ta.

Re-reading this I too wonder, was this the homework you were set? Probably not, but this short extract from your journal notes illustrates how education will out. Therapists set homework, but the patient will have experiences regardless. The original reflection on 'bigness' and its potential downside drew you to reflect on something that you think might be an enduring dimension of your character – your need for others: being a 'people person'. Ironically, you begin to trace a deep vein of weakness – as you seem to see it – from the vantage point of a peak experience. There you were, sitting in the bath, experiencing a veritable rush of 'new ideas', and you felt your boundaries stretching and didn't want the stretching to stop. However, mulling it all over, that joyous chain of events left you realizing that you *needed* some control, some discipline, although you did not actually *want* this. You didn't want this because the joy of discovery was proving to be too much fun. Maybe I should have asked you what you would have *wished* for.

A powerful temptation exists, to *interpret* your descent from the high plateau of enthusiasm with which you began this extract to the creeping doubts that ended the note twenty lines later. Indeed, you begin to dive into such interpretations yourself before fielding them out to me for confirmation or criticism. Such interpretations are the stuff (if not the nonsense) of classical psychotherapy. The traditional therapist would likely doze gently through the early stage of your account (you are just too positive to be interesting), but would likely pounce lustfully on the last few lines. Here lies the therapists's 'ah-hah' experience. Here lies the evidence that might confirm his hypothesis as to what (exactly) was going on behind that cleverly woven story of growth and development. Here lies *his* story rather than *her* story! Do you really want me to interpret this? There doesn't seem to be any need, as you seem to be doing fine all by yourself.

There is just enough wondering going on in your narrative to suggest to me that your life is rolling along quite nicely. You are beginning to develop the kind of appreciation of 'self' that David Reynolds holds so well (or badly, depending on one's ideological position). You simply haven't yet acquired his almost phlegmatic acceptance that life is to be experienced, not predicted; and certainly not on the basis of past events and past behaviour[4].

---

[4]It is worth noting here that Reynolds has written often about his fear of flying. In his view, this is just part of who he is – not something that needs to be treated or fixed or somehow got rid of. Rather, it is a part of who he is that requires him to 'do what needs to be done', to somehow live with, through or (perhaps even) transcend such an experience. Many of Reynolds' students are the fortunate recipients of flower paintings, which he does on long flights. In Reynolds' view, life is meant to be lived – not necessarily free from anxiety, or pain or any other human distress. The primary focus needs to be on living constructively – peeling potatoes, dusting a bookcase or weeding a patch of garden, not as a distraction from feelings, but because we have decided that these are the things that *need* doing, even when we don't necessarily want to do them. Of course, when we lose ourselves in such activities we may experience a lessening of distressing feelings, but that is not the primary objective, just an interesting way-station.

Suddenly it all makes sense

Monday, August 24 12.20 am

I just quit watching a Jack Lemmon movie called Mass Appeal, *and now I want to talk to you. The bit that really got to me was right near the end when Jack Lemmon says he thought he needed the love of his congregation and he was afraid of losing. His young protegé, who got kicked out by the hierarchy because he didn't conform, said that to really love you have to be prepared to risk losing. That's what I'll call a 'that's it in a nutshell'. Do you ever get those? It's what happens when you've been half aware of something going around the back corridors of the brain, and suddenly out it comes through the front door into the light, crystal clear.*

Earlier today I was having a talk with F, who is torn between encouraging her children's independence and feeling threatened by their reduced need for her. My feeling stronger has risks too. Now, looking back, I think I was holding on to my weakness because 'getting better' would mean I was out on my own. Very risky. Getting my confidence back, starting to deal with things, makes that seem imminent. That is scary. I think what's good is that I accept that. I'm not sure what to do about the scary bit, but I know I don't want to go back to the 'safety' of stagnation. I'm opting for the unknown and taking a bet that's a risk worth taking.

I took a drive in the late afternoon, just to sit in the sun for an hour and read a bit of one of the books you'd recommended. I had been feeling a bit dubious about our meeting on Thursday, because I hadn't done the homework you set. There was a time when I would have been terrified that you would be angry, but I know you better now and have no such fears. Still, I did think you'd probably be disappointed in me, and I don't like to disappoint you. From the outset, I was unclear what the homework was. My thinking is the reason I couldn't remember what you asked me to do was that it didn't immediately 'click' with me. It didn't fit into my own thought patterns about what I need to do. No ideas popped into my head as you were speaking, so there was nothing to fix it in my head. Now that was my thinking. Today, while I'm reading a textbook, it seems to be saying the same thing a bit differently. It says the therapist should make sure the client understands the instructions for homework, or he won't be able to carry them out successfully. Another 'that's it in a nutshell'. I should've made it clear to you I wasn't grasping what I was supposed to do.

The communication breakdown, having affected my ability to do homework, meant I was concerned you would perceive my non-productiveness as lack of effort and motivation on my part. I have been reading a little bit of the textbooks every day to demonstrate willingness, but now I'm not so sure you will be pleased with that. I was reading about interview techniques today, and I kept saying to myself, 'So that's why he asks that or does that'. Now I'm thinking you'll probably be concerned about me reading because I might start being aware of the techniques more than what we're saying. Do you think being aware of a problem, or a potential problem, is half way to solving it? I need to believe that, because so often all I seem to be able to do is articulate the problem but not know how to tackle it right off.

That journal entry reminds me of how you were beginning to focus on particular world views – your belief systems, rather than just the individual life problems that you had brought with you to therapy. This entry is, like the others in this chapter, from the later stages, and illustrates the timeliness of dealing with world views as and when they push themselves to the centre stage of therapy and not before. If we had tried to deal with these bigger picture issues earlier, the canvas of your understanding (so to speak) might have buckled under all the painted detail we would (of necessity) have been applying.

Reflecting on your original question reminds me of how reasonable it is to assume that people act on their beliefs and their lives roll out as a dramatization of those individual little acts. The history of human achievement and failure, social order and disorder, and the propagation of good and evil, all seem to pivot around particular beliefs – world views, if you like. You were relating to a specific world view that 'being aware of a problem is half way to solving it.' That seemed to work for you, in the sense that it met some need in you. That doesn't mean of course that it is the *right* view – generally true for others. That is the curse of normalcy; the notion that there are right and wrong ways to live one's life. The English comedian Harry Enfield portrays an interfering yet neighbourly character who is always sticking his nose into others' business, telling them 'you don't wanna be doing that, you should be doing ...' (something else). Enfield's character is so inoffensively dressed – in bowling cap, neat golfing jersey and horn-rimmed spectacles – that he epitomizes Middle England and conformity. The character belies, however, a darker side. Such inoffensiveness disguises the oppression held within simple words like 'should' and 'must'. These are the moral imperatives drilled into us as children by earnest, often well-meaning, parents and teachers. Unlike Enfield's cheerily irritating character, these childhood influences shape our adult neuroses – especially the need for social approval and acceptance.

Once, when running an experiential workshop, I 'role played' a character who dipped down into his childhood self and drew out an experience of being told 'don't do that, people won't like you'. I used the experience to illustrate to the group that what 'it' was did not really matter. Rather, the moral instruction contained in the phrasing '... people won't like you', would (likely) be sufficient to instil a fear of rejection in the child-as-adult. As I developed this theoretical point with group, the realization dawned that the childhood character I had 'developed' was none other than myself. I would be trivializing the whole complex business of being a child and becoming adult if I suggested that my non-conformist nature and lifestyle is entirely a function of the *happening* on that childhood day. I would, however, be disingenuous if I suggested that it played no part in shaping the *me* whom *I* have become[5].

I note that, having read my view that the therapist should ensure that the patient understands the point of any homework, you decided to take that responsibility upon yourself. Perhaps 'excusing the teacher' is something that you picked up somewhere down the earlier days of your life. Certainly, it can be popular with all sorts of people who have a responsibility for instilling values or ideas. When they fail to pass across this piece of learning, they can attribute it to the student's failure to pick it up. I smiled when I re-read that point, for clearly I do not always take my own good advice. You have reminded me – paradoxically – that although you define and re-define yourself, it remains my responsibility to help you to appreciate your own power for personal good or ill. That, perhaps, is the therapist's challenge, 'in a nutshell', and a pretty big nutshell it can be.

Speaking of good advice, much of your reflections on 'doing and being' and the whole business of the joy of discovery remind me of Confucius, who was alleged to have said:

> Young people should be good sons at home, polite and respectful in society, careful in their conduct and faithful. They should love the people, and associate themselves with the kind people. If after learning all this they still have the energy, *let them read books*.

This is a form of wisdom that is rapidly escaping us as we wed ourselves more and more to 'concepts', especially the strangely modern concept of self-concept, 'Who do I think *I* am?' The Chinese sage Chaung Tzu had quite a different set of 'shoulds and musts' from those popularized by the Protestant ethic. Chaung Tzu affirmed that 'you should cherish that which is within you, and shut off that which is without – for much knowledge is a curse'. Lin-Chi had yet another simple set of affirmations: 'when hungry, eat your rice, when tired, close your eyes. Fools may laugh at me, but wise men will know what I mean'. Clearly these men (if indeed they were individuals and not a whole philosophical tradition) had little idea that two millennia later we might look back so fondly on their simple words of such simple truth. As we enter the third millennium we are not only 'hung up' on the neuroses fostered by

---

[5]Albert Ellis developed a highly innovative form of humanistic therapy called Rational Emotive Therapy (RET), which focused on challenging the Irrational Beliefs that Ellis believed generated emotional distress. Ellis' therapeutic style was often highly irreverent. He popularized the idea of giving patients 'homework assignments', and would encourage groups of patients to sing specially written songs describing their anxieties, woes or fears, to the tune of *Yankee Doodle Dandy*.

parent–child dynamics, but have also cultivated new ways to be neurotic. Our information age has bred information anxiety – the fear that we might miss something that we *should* know about. Perhaps we no longer believe, as Socrates did, that all that we can be certain of is our own ignorance – or, as Huxley observed, who can be considered out of danger, if a little knowledge is a dangerous thing? True, this is an information age, but is information knowledge?

Don Juan suggested that the more one seduces the less one loves. Perhaps, the more we are informed, the less we know. Less often is more. The information that we ingest (but rarely digest) becomes a part of us. What we choose to read and choose to ignore, therefore, has critical implications for who we, ultimately, become. However, often such decisions are made arbitrarily, as if such experiences will not exact any significant influence on who we become. There are some indications here of you picking and choosing from different sources of information, weighing these carefully in terms of their potential contribution to the emergent 'you'. This is significant in the light of the recent fashion for explaining things to patients – such as their illness and their experience. Whereas Freud believed in the 'psychopathology of everyday life', many therapists are today keen to reframe meaningful experiences of a disturbing world as *psychopathology* — teaching their patients to use the language of medicine or psychology to frame their experience. Another example, perhaps of the psychiatric power-game articulated so well by Foucault (1988).

Monday December 9

Last night I discovered something really important in your book (Barker, 1992). I'm talking about p. 232, where you are introducing common unhelpful thoughts which trouble depressed people. The important bit for me is, 'It is worth noting that they trouble most people, but they trouble depressed people more seriously'. It was one of those statements which, when seen in black and white, seems blindingly obvious, but I hadn't previously articulated it for myself. I have never thought I was depressed, but it has troubled me in a way that such a lot of the book makes sense to me and I can relate the content to direct personal experience. A stupid fear of being classed as a real 'nutter' underlies that, I think. Right from the start, even I understood that at some level my problem was my experience and my understanding of the world, which was quite severely disabling my function in the world. The point is that everyone has unhelpful thoughts, but people find ways of coping which prevents them being disabling – or reduces the level of disability. We have been hugely successful at damage limitation. Well, I think we have.

You will recall that it was around this time that we began to focus on 'meditation in life'. I guess that, having spent a lot of time examining and exploring your experience, it was time to arrange some conditions that might allow you to experience some different experiences. It had always been clear that you were aware of your *self*. Now seemed as good a time as any to explore awareness *for its own sake*. This was where discipline entered the script. Up until then your homework had been largely done inside your head – often involving a deeper appreciation of 'getting confused', as you have noted before. When you begin to think about what you think, and explore what, exactly, you believe about what you believe, inevitably some confusion emerges. But confusion is good, if only as a reflection of something that just 'is' – that is, your experience.

The experience of other forms of 'just being' gradually occupied more and more of the therapeutic agenda. Some might argue that we should have done more of this stuff earlier, as you patently found it to be of such benefit, and it was so simple. But it was neither simple, nor simply something that can be slotted into the daily programme of someone who isn't exactly sure if they are a real 'nutter' or not. The very fact that you conjured with such questions about your identity suggested, to me at least, that the meditation in life came at just about the right time – when you had largely passed over such heavily socially conditioned fears about your own everyday madness.

But I should not continue without considering your rhetorical question as to what, exactly, a 'real nutter' might be, and whether you ever were – even transiently – worthy of the label 'true madness'. I confess that this is a question which has long exercised me, though not in quite the way that you perhaps frame it. Psychiatry has a long tradition of separating the crazy person, the lunatic and the insane from those possessed of more ordinary forms of madness. I tend to agree with my wise old friend Tom Szasz, that all such classification with its 'terms like neurosis, psychosis, mental illness, indeed the whole gamut of psychiatric diagnostic labels, functions mainly as counters in a pseudomedical rhetoric of rejection' (Szasz, 1971). Indeed, you may have been trying to distance yourself from the 'truly mad' (the real nutter) – a version of the kind of rejection that Tom Szasz sees as integral to the whole psychiatric classification system.

I feel a deep sadness that, after 2000 years of appreciation of 'madness' (beginning with the Greeks) and more than 200 years of modern psychiatric medicine, we still try to separate people from their experience. True, we allow people with minor problems involving the self to muse endlessly with their therapists on their putative meaning – the Woody Allen scenario. However, those who enact more dramatic scenarios risk being dispossessed entirely of their right to muse, in any way, on their possible human significance, unless of course they do this for and by themselves – which, increasingly, many people are doing (Barker *et al.*, 1999). There is, of course, a long tradition of reflecting on madness by poets and authors, many of whom were (from time to time) patently mad, crazy or insane. The list would include your favourite poet, William

Blake. We may take our pick of the rejecting epithets. I, however, cannot but marvel at the way some of these people have recovered their identity, rising like a phoenix from the ashes of their experience (Barker, 1998).

It seems that madness is an experience of something that tells the person she has somehow gone over the edge, or lost the plot of her life. Once, all forms of social deviation risked being defined as madness (Foucault, 1988). Recently, we have returned to the naturalistic approach of trying to put different forms of madness in boxes, discriminating (often for dubious political reasons) between the 'seriously and enduringly mentally ill' (Barker *et al.*, 1999) and (presumably) people who are only 'trivially mentally ill'. Although people's lives can be brought to a sudden halt by anxiety, as you are aware, this risks beings dismissed as a trivial mental health problem. I never thought that your problems were 'trivial', although clearly you were not what would be called, in the common parlance, a 'real nutter'. Such distinctions miss the point. When the New Zealand author Janet Frame wrote of her own slide into an apparently inexorable madness, she appreciated the need – like you – to write (Frame, 1980):

> I shall write about the season of peril. I was put in hospital because a great gap opened in the ice floe between myself and other people whom I watched, with their world drifting away through a violet-coloured sea where hammer-headed sharks in tropical ease swam side by side with the seals and polar bears. I was alone on the ice.

Leaving aside the lyrical yet fearsome beauty of her reflections, this is a woman who is becoming acutely aware of her self and what it might mean to be Janet Frame. She continued:

> But the shop windows were speaking to me, and the rain too, running down inside the window of the fish shop, and the clean moss and fern inside the florists, and the dowdy droopy two-piece sets and old-fashioned coats hung on aged plaster models in the cheaper shops that could not afford to light their windows ... They all spoke. They said Beware of the Sale, Beware of the Bargain Prices. Beware of traffic and germs; if you find a handkerchief hold it up by the tip of the finger and thumb until it is claimed. For a cold in the chest be steamed with Friar's Balsam. Do not sit on the seat of public lavatory. Danger. Power lines overhead.

> I was not yet civilized; I traded my safety for the glass beads of fantasy.

Somehow people like Janet Frame recovered their balance, perhaps returning the glass beads of fantasy in the process and accepting the insecurity of the water-tormented world in which she saw her own many faces.

The final ascent

Wednesday, September 2 10 pm

I shall miss you, but I am not afraid. Most of what I need is in myself. If I keep looking I will find it. Thank you for guiding me through the foothills. We are almost at the base of the mountain, and when we reach it I shall say goodbye and not look back. My face will turn up to the summit. Thank you for preparing me for the climb ...

I remember when I gave the counsellor my brother's copy of Blake. He cried and cried. I was afraid. I didn't understand. Now I can read his letter from that time and understand that he put a different value on that gift. He saw it as some sort of turning point in the relationship. I gave him a spare copy of a book because I wanted him to read the book and hear what I was hearing in the words. But the value he placed on it was as an object that had belonged to my beloved brother. I doubt he has ever read any of the poems.

As you begin your final ascent I note that you do not promise to look back, but perhaps that is only at me. You do manage a look back at the counsellor and the analyst and, from your new vantage point, see things quite differently. Now that might seem predictable, but it *is* interesting. I suppose what you wrote here is a version of the old saying, 'one day you'll look back on this and laugh'. Of course, most of us want that day to be as close as possible – if not right now. However, the really interesting thing is what happens between now and that day in the future which folk wisdom knows will allow us to 'look back in laughter'.

I appreciate that it is difficult to establish an endpoint. Really this is because there is no such thing. I remember telling you once that when I stopped evolving I would die. My experience of therapy is that it has brought me to an awareness of my evolution. Since the evolving is continuous, there is no endpoint. But of course our relationship must find a conclusion. How and when I can't answer. I gain from being with you, but I also know I wouldn't stop gaining from not being with you. The answer is probably that someone else needs your time more. But I am selfish!

It is exactly seven years to the day since you wrote those lines, as I begin to wrap up my reflections on your journals and draw this chapter to a close, perhaps trying to find an echo of Leonardo in my own clumsy metaphors. Our relationship has gone through several incarnations since you stepped out of the artificial illumination of therapy into the natural light of your own life. I have little idea of how you have changed over those years, but I am reassured that the joy of discovery – which we selected originally as the title for this penultimate chapter – still seems like valid currency. I guess you might find it hard to summarize succinctly what exactly happened between the afternoon of your first appointment and that moment when you found you had the freedom to 'look back in laughter' (or, more correctly, wisdom). Perhaps you said it yourself, you became more aware of yourself and, as Thoreau said, it is as hard to see one's self as to look backwards without turning around. Now that you are looking back (literally and metaphorically) through these journals, maybe you can see more clearly. Such is the logic of experience.

Your observation that the endpoint doesn't exist is a fitting end in itself. It doesn't exist, so we have to construct one. This, the root of the issue, reminds me of the story of the man who began to lose his hair. It got thinner and thinner until he had only one hair left, which he combed and brushed and shampooed carefully each day. One morning he awoke to find the hair on his pillow. The man was distraught; 'my God,' he cried, 'I'm bald!' Life is summed up neatly in that story. Things come on so gradually. Change threads its way so seamlessly through our lives, that to ask 'when did things begin to change?' is a silly question. Change is something we wake up to.

References

Barker, P. (1992). *Severe Depression: A Practitioner's Guide*. Chapman and Hall.
Barker, P. (1998). Creativity and psychic distress in writers, artists and scientists. *Journal of Psychiatric and Mental Health Nursing*, **5**(2), 109–18.
Barker, P., Campbell, P. and Davidson, B. (eds) (1999). *From the Ashes of Experience: Reflections on Madness, Recovery and Growth*. Whurr.
Ellis, A. (1962). *Reason and Emotion in Psychotherapy*. Lyle and Stuart.
Foucault, M. (1988). *Madness and Civilization*. Vintage.
Frame, J. (1980). *Faces in the Water*. The Women's Press.
Kopp, S. (1978). *If You meet the Buddha on the Road, Kill Him!* Sheldon Press.
Machiavelli, N. (1961). *The Prince* (trans. G. Bull). Penguin.
Reynolds, D. (1985). *Playing Ball on Running Water*. Sheldon Press.
Reynolds, D. (1987). *The Sound of Rippling Water: Constructive Living through Morita and Naikan Therapies*. (Audiocassette)
Szasz, T. (1971). *Ideology and Insanity*, p. 60. Penguin.
Turner, R. (1993). *Inventing Leonardo: The Anatomy of a Legend*. Papermac.

9

The road to nowhere

Well we know where we're going
But we don't know where we've been
And we know what we're knowing
But we can't say what we've seen

And we're not little children
And we know what we want
For the future is certain
Give us time to work it out

David Byrne

The road to somewhere

The last formal correspondence between therapist and patient took place in February. As I was preparing my formal report on the outcome of the therapy, I asked you to prepare an 'alternative report'. It seemed appropriate. What had you made of the encounters?

You submitted your report promptly, and it seemed – at one and the same time – to be both spontaneous and highly considered. Maybe you simply committed your 'felt knowledge' to paper. I was envious.

That kind of knowledge seemed more interesting than the various measures of 'patient satisfaction' and 'clinical outcome' with which I was struggling, and which had become, even six or seven years ago, the stuff (if not the nonsense) of a service driven increasingly by economic rationalism. Your report was also far more revealing of yourself and of the value of our therapeutic relationship. It lies somewhere at the core of all our current ruminations about the quality of care and treatment and human services, that we seem to be talking now about a monetarist value. You, on the other hand, seemed to be trying to take stock of the value of a special kind of human encounter that might almost be virtuous – by virtue of what happened for both parties. That you dealt so simply with the meaning of the encounter was the main grounds for my envy, given that I was meant to be the articulate one, if not also the articulator of meaning.

Today, on the cusp of the millennium, many might take the view that I dedicated too much of my time to untried and untested clinical techniques. You might now be advised, through some glossy patient information leaflet, that your needs would have been better served by a therapist who had focused on a more straightforward course of 'psycho-education' about the nature of anxiety and depression, the psychological sequelae of past traumatic experience, and more direct tutelage in the various methods of 'managing anxiety'. Although arguably some of this received wisdom was part of our encounter, I opened out the therapeutic canvas to allow you to access a wider range of possible forms of human helpfulness. To a great extent we made it up as we went along; such is the nature of interpersonal relations. I never had any doubts that I was trying to respond to you as a person, rather than as a patient, and was adapting myself, session by session, in an effort better to meet your needs. I learned a lot about the business of therapy, if not also myself, in the process. So I had to conclude that the overall outcome was a success. However, my main yardstick was that you seemed no longer to *need* the therapy. Your 'alternative report' reinforced my utilitarian judgement, and concurred with that judgement. The case was about to close, but the story of the casework was still very much open.

A reflection

Dear Phil

Many years ago I discovered the enclosed 'therapeutic gift'[1]. Last Thursday, you asked me how I felt about 'discharge'. If you listen to Hesse, he will tell you where we are standing on the road to nowhere (Hesse, 2000):

> As every flower fades and as all youth
> Departs, so life at every stage,
> So every virtue, so our grasp of truth,
> Blooms in its day and may not last forever.
> Since life may summon us at every age

---

[1] Earlier, we had talked about how various writers offered, often unwittingly, 'therapeutic gifts' in the form of their writings.

Be ready, heart, for parting, new endeavour,
Be ready bravely and without remorse
To find new light that old ties cannot give.
In all beginnings dwells a magic force
For guarding us and helping us to live.

Serenely let us move to distant places
And let no sentiments of home detain us.
The Cosmic Spirit seeks not to restrain us
But lifts us stage by stage to wider spaces.
If we accept a home of our own making,
Familiar habit makes for indolence.
We must prepare for parting and leave taking
Or else remain the slaves of permanence.

Even the hour of our death may send
Us speeding on to fresh and newer spaces,
And life may summon us to newer races,
So be it, heart: bid farewell without end.

Regarding my discharge letter, I feel 'Phil is brill' would just about cover what I want to say, but it doesn't sound very doctoral, does it? The following seems reasonable.

Bobbie has moved from being a person overwhelmed by everyday living and paralysed by the fear of what could happen to her or those she holds dear, to being a person who eagerly participates in ordinary living and keeps open to unexpected joys and opportunities.

She is now confident in her ability to cope with future disappointments and tragedies, but is not paralysed by anticipation of such events.

She has gained enormous benefit from the practical techniques she has learned, which reduced her initial distress and gave her an awareness of stress factors, stress reactions, and her own ability to control these.

Bobbie states that the greatest benefit has come from the patient attention of her therapist, who forged a relationship within which she gained her trust in others, herself and the world.

Thanks hardly seems adequate.

Bobbie

Stories, stories and more stories

I was impressed by your 'signing-off' from the therapeutic engagement, the first time I read it. If you prick us do we not bleed? as the Bard wisely put it, and if you tickle the therapist does he not laugh? – at least inwardly, with satisfaction. Although therapists have long been coached in the virtue of dampening their emotional reactivity, this tradition, borne of the ideology of psychoanalysis, has less and less currency – at least in my book. Therapy is an interpersonal encounter, and requires at least two fully functioning humans to make the necessary psychic sparks fly. We have known that since Harry Stack Sullivan first began to map his appreciation of what was going on *between* him and the patient (Sullivan, 1953), and Frieda Fromm Reichman sat down on the floor with the patient, expressing a desire to *join with* the person (Fromm Reichman, 1950). Both were trying to escape from the limitations of the crude notion that therapists could somehow see into the souls as well as minds of patients without actually making contact with the ground, from which such metaphysical dimensions of the self sprung. Re-reading your goodbye instils a different feeling seven years later, but it is still a pleasurable one. My pleasure at your satisfaction with the relationship that we forged seems wholly appropriate, despite the concerns of several generations of therapists that we should feel uncomfortable about obtaining overt pleasure from the labours of the therapeutic process. This may simply signal another departure point for me from the traditional boundaries of the psychotherapy trade.

Stated most simply and boldly, as I have said repeatedly, psychotherapy is just two people talking – one harbouring the intention to be helpful towards the other. I would be lying if I even suggested that I brought any less than my whole life experience to the therapeutic encounter. Some of that experience was formed in encounters with patients like you, but much more came from that fickle teacher, the University of Life. I am lucky to have led a fortunate life, full of drama and eventfulness. The sheer unpredicatability of my fortunate life has been my greatest teacher[2]. I hope that I brought some of the lessons, painfully learned there, to the therapeutic encounter.

All of which simply affirms that therapists bring to the therapeutic conversation their own meanings, which is why I have tried to explicate my own meanings in this book. I shall say some more in this conclusion about the vexed business of 'being helpful' in a moment. Here I want to comment on the way you reframed that simple process elegantly when you noted that the relationship we forged to allow that conversation to develop helped you to develop the capacity to trust not only yourself – no mean feat – but also others and the world. How could I not be pleased? I would, however, draw the line at flattery.

---

[2]An old friend in New Zealand once described how we had both led 'fortunate lives'. Two days later in Sydney, another friend made a gift of Albert Facey's autobiography, *A Fortunate Life*. In that remarkable book, Facey – who had been illiterate for most of his life – described his journey from survival in Gallipoli to the writing of a bestseller at the age of 87 years. Having written about life *as if* it were a journey, Albert Facey has been rightly described as 'Australia's pilgrim' (Facey, 1985).

For I need to confess my understanding (again) of what I believe happened within that relationship, where we found ourselves talking to such good effect. The relationship allowed you to access and explore some of the more significant pages of your story – your narrative, if you like. There, you began to edit or re-author some of the assertions and assumptions you had made previously about your *self*, and how that self operated in the world of your emerging experience. It may not entirely be true that knowledge of history will prevent us repeating our mistakes. Ignorance of who we have been, however, as well as a lack of awareness of who we are now, will certainly have some implications for the 'who' we shall soon become. Such is the destiny project.

It may be noteworthy that this book – or rather the conversation that has been fleshed out to form the book – emerged from your journals. Those journals expressed your natural desire to signal something of your experience of 'me' to the 'I' who often caught glimmers of understanding about what Bobbie Kerr was experiencing. Although these signals were developed into a form of reporting to me (the 'other'), their audience, first and foremost, was your own self: the 'I' who is the 'me' of Bobbie.

Although it is true that all therapy involves storytelling, not all patients appreciate the significance of the unfolding narrative. Or rather, they do not necessarily appreciate the extent to which each act of recording their story – even as breath into the air of the consulting room – signals that editing process to which I refer. That sounds patronizing, doesn't it? However, I fear that this personal ignorance is manufactured in part by our consumerist society, and in part by the psychotherapy trade itself. Psychotherapy has become a means more of fixing people than of understanding them and, by implication, aiding their self-understanding. Increasingly, therapy is less about change and more about adjustment. Perhaps too many people have come to believe that therapists actively 'adjust' them, when the human reality may be that therapists are merely a necessary presence to the process of self-adjustment.

Yet people do make themselves up as they talk, as my old mentor Hildegard E. Peplau (1910–99) used to say. When that talk is rendered in physical form, like your journal, it assumes not just a new form but also a new significance. Traditional psychiatric (and often psychotherapeutic) practice involves taking a *his*-tory. This is a story whose boundaries and content are largely determined by the therapist. The control (often) lies in his hands. Hence the feminist's argument in favour of *her*-story as an alternative: a story that provides a balance to the masculine perspective on the world. What emerged in our relationship was a fairly swift shift from any emphasis on the taking of a psychiatric or therapeutic history to a focus on your appreciation of the importance of *her*-story: Bobbie's tale, its content and its meaning. In the process, something of the *mystery* of your disabling experience was clarified. If you like, the his-tory that became her-story finally became my-story, as you embraced the re-authored narrative. Of course, in re-authoring your story (the original my-story) you made no attempt to overwrite the 'bad bits', but simply cast them in a different light. Perhaps that is a form of everyday enlightenment. Towards the end of the encounter I saw more and more signs of that 'enlightenment'.

I've been trying to put a distance between myself and all this pretence for a couple of weeks – that is, there's no real hassle, nothing I can't handle. Well, at the end of the day I suppose that's true, but it is not realized or achieved by ignoring what I'm thinking or feeling.

The thing that gets me is here I am trying to be positive and develop helpful attitudes and often, in the midst of my big thinks, all I am really certain of is how uncertain I am about anything. I think I've got something or someone sussed and adopt a helpful attitude, and then for no apparent reason that changes.

But maybe this is all there is. Maybe that's what you're trying to help me do – realize that there are no absolute responses when faced with certain situations. Just go with the flow and adopt what seems the right response at the time, even if that's different from the last time. And nothing is completely the same, is it?

And later you began to draw together some threads from your recollection of your time spent with the analyst and the counsellor:

With both A and C I felt trapped in my terrors. I came to feel I needed the therapist, but felt that they needed me to stay with the terrors. It is so complicated. With both of them I would come out of a session terrorized and exhausted, yet I couldn't drag myself away from that and say it wasn't working for me. I felt they were the only people I could really be with, although the sessions were obviously frustrating and unsatisfactory for both of us. I didn't feel there was anywhere to go if I left. There was no way for me to exist except in this overly dependent, frustrating 'relationship'. Because, I think, I had no vision of where to go, I was afraid to leave, afraid to get 'well'. Does this make sense?

I remember saying to you latterly, after you said to me a door was opening for me, that I felt scores of doors were there to be opened and I wanted to go through them all and I was unafraid of what might be behind them. I think that is when I knew I was truly well.

This door metaphor suggests something of the turnaround you had accomplished – or perhaps simply become aware of. You moved from a position where doors were, effectively, closed to you, to one where there were many doors waiting to be opened. Paradoxically, the proliferation of options and choices that once would have fazed you now provides a source of delight. This suggested to me the beginning of an appreciation of a sense of internal connectedness: the beginnings of 'Possibility Land' (O'Hanlon and Beadle, 1997).

Having drawn the line earlier at flattery, I may flatter myself by assuming that this meant that I had given you a 'good hearing' as well as a 'fair listening'. The therapist is audience as well as performer, and needs to engage with the actor, who is temporarily cast in the role of patient. However, the patient – as well as the society that ultimately foots the bill – assumes that the therapist is the actor at the centre of the stage, spewing wise words, even if the wisdom is not entirely his own. This actor analogy reminds me of Brian Cox, an actor who grew up in Dundee (the town where I first trained) and who reflected on his performance of King Lear to the patients at Broadmoor Special Hospital. Cox was talking about how London audiences, on the whole, don't deal well with challenging performances, but want to be reassured. In Cox's view, Shakespeare could 'always be dressed up as wonderful poetry, or wonderful music, or something which has an aesthetic about it, though it also has hard dealings with human behaviour. But they [the London audiences] do not like that kind of Shakespeare, they love the lyrical, they always love the poetic. They don't realize where the poetry comes from' (Cox, 1992). Cox went on to talk about how he sensed the Broadmoor audience bringing those 'hard dealings' from him:

> They brought it out more than any other audience … In a way, I am more interested in an audience's reactions than I am in what we do for audiences. I want to see what they get out of it, as opposed to what we get out of it. I think it is very important to understand what an audience experiences; it does not matter whether it is an audience of mad people, or an audience of sane people. What is actually happening in that process, what is the whole act of sitting watching something about? What is actually going on when you watch? Because it can't be just purely about entertainment, it has to be something about expiation. It has to be something which is about taking sins away from you.

Although we often do not attribute wisdom to actors, these are wise words indeed. The enactment of therapy that took place between us involved a play on the words of your story, intermingling this with some of what it meant for me as well as for you. The story that unfolded was a live one in the sense that Cox recognizes the play is always live, since it involves the audience actively whether they want to engage or not. I am sure that a similar kind of engagement occurred with the analyst and the counsellor, but maybe the rules of engagement were different, and so what you (the audience/actor) took away from it was different. Like Brian Cox, for a long time I have been more interested in what the patient makes of my performance rather than my performance itself. Maybe I find my role in getting lost in the audience reaction.

The subtleties of the power relationship

What I took away from our last meeting was your statement to one of your students that the therapist must work really hard in the beginning, then in the later stages the patient takes over and does most of the work on her own. It's like it happens in the presence of the therapist rather than something the therapist makes happen. In my head I have two pictures. One is of us both at sea in a ferocious storm, and you are at the helm using all your strength just to keep the boat from crashing into the rocks and breaking up. The other is of us both becalmed in a little open boat, and I am sitting talking to you and every so often, almost imperceptibly, you gently guide the tiller.

I can't remember if I have talked to you before about encouraging a vision of the future, but if I have, I think it's such an important idea it bears repeating. In the beginning (most certainly in my case) the therapist has to work very hard just to find a piece of safe ground for us to meet on. He has a monumental task to show me it is safe to let him in. But later, after most of the barriers have been overcome, there is a big danger this relationship becomes such a safe place to be − I am scared to get 'too well' because then I lose the relationship and the safe place. Of course, the antidote to that is a positive vision of the future.

You gave me the confidence to create a positive vision of the future. I became excited about all the possibilities of my life, and wanted (and still want) to rush about doing exciting, fulfilling things. Most helpfully, I learned that relationships do change, this is their very nature, but I learned not to be threatened by that. Yes, it is sad when someone who has played a big part in your life becomes less important, less involved, but it makes way for something new, something different, instead of a desperate clinging to what is fading away. In my experience, desperate clinging is the last strangling that completely kills what is left.

That note read as another signal for Possibility Land. I guess in the beginning you might have been keen to cling to any old wreckage, but in time you found that desperate clinging is the last thing you want or even need. At the risk of sounding falsely modest, maybe that time was the important gift. All too often, the message we give to people is 'be like this for me ... do this for me'. Wittingly or unwittingly, we want people to be like us, to conform to our ideas of 'right' and 'wrong', of the 'good life'. We want them to take on our identity, and so we end up *territorializing* them, recasting them in our image and likeness. I would be lying if I said I hadn't ever operated in that kind of way in both my private and professional life, but now I hope I know better. Now I hope that I am happy to encounter people like you, and to be genuinely interested in what you *make* of your life and of me. That kind of encounter might involve the 'gift of time'.

Traditional therapy (especially when cast within the province of psychiatry) territorializes people, often unwittingly. Therapists talk, casually, of 'my patient' or 'a patient of mine', as if the person had become a professional property. Although this desire to territorialize (and therefore dominate) people is threaded through our social hierarchies and contracts, it lies at the heart of the professional conspiracy against the laity, as Shaw defined it[3]. What you gained from our encounter was not something that I specifically set up for you. I had no ambition to shape you in one form or another, to guide you in one direction or another. I was keen to see what you might *make* of the encounter and, in that very specific sense, how you might *reconstruct* yourself. Your conclusion that I gave you confidence is interesting, since that was not something I was consciously offering. It makes a fitting conclusion to hear that you found what you needed (or wanted) in the gift of my time[4,5]

Defining and finding health

If this project has involved you in clarifying further what *actually* happened in the therapeutic process, for me it has involved a significant chapter in the story of my deconstruction as a therapist. In my attempts to return to the simple vocation that brought me into health care and psychotherapy in the first place, I discover that such places no longer exist – or exist only in my memory. They have been replaced by a professional landscape, which is more concerned with developing a body of knowledge (research) *about* people than it is concerned with the facilitation of self-knowledge[6]. Even my primary discipline (nursing) has forsaken its vocation, to the great regret of some nurses (Inglesby, 1992):

> When a candidate is asked at interview why she [*sic*] chose nursing, the correct answer is no longer 'I want to help people'. ... The value upon care remains high, but care is no longer 'tender' or 'loving', it is a specifiable commodity ... A nurse is no longer dedicated; she is professional. She is no longer moral; she is accountable.

---

[3]Although it is a hackneyed critique, we need to remind ourselves that the professional language of psychiatry (and psychotherapy) was designed to keep the layperson at a distance, if not in the dark, and perforce dependent.

[4]Derrida has written about the 'true gift' as something that one does not realize one is giving. Since such a gift is not based on any notion of reciprocity ('I'll give you this if ...'), Derrida believed it had the capacity to deterritorialize (Derrida, 1992).

[5]It is apparent that professionals, especially those who see their work as a vocation, often pretend to give *freely* of themselves when, in effect, the giving is characterized by reciprocity – especially the expectation that the recipient will be grateful, or even simply will acknowledge the effort expended. Professional gifts can be like outward shows of 'godliness', where the superiority of the therapist is defined, perhaps with a view to storing up credits for a therapeutic after-life (Mauss, 1990; Fox, 1999). Although gift-like, these acts of giving can be seen as acts of aggression, involving an exposure of the weakness of the other (Moi, 1985).

[6]This concern extends across the spectrum of the helping professions (see Shrock, 1982).

Perhaps naively, I still cling to the romantic fiction that I might be of help to people, maybe through the empty 'gift of time'.

Now that you believe yourself to be well implies that once you were *unwell* – perhaps even *ill* or *sick*. This illustrates further the importance of metaphor, since I don't think that you were *sick* in anything other than a 'sick at heart' or 'soul sick' sense. I doubt if you did either. We could say that you had recovered from whatever it was that had ailed you, but that also is problematic. Writing about her 'recovery' from what had been called a chronic psychosis, Sally Clay wrote (Clay, 1999):

> … but if I have recovered, what have I recovered from, and what have I recovered to?

Sally preferred to construe her situation differently. After many years of disabling 'psychotic breakdowns', involving repeated, damaging hospitalizations, Sally concluded that she had '… not recovered. I have *overcome*'. Perhaps your 'getting well' involved a similar kind of 'overcoming'.

Many people who read this book will, of course, approach the notion of 'getting well' and 'being ill' from a different perspective. For some, whatever it was that 'ailed' you would not be a metaphorical thing so much as a real *ailment* (if a minor illness) or *disorder* (if a more serious one). They would want to know what was *wrong* with Bobbie. It is not only professionals who have become preoccupied with diagnoses and classifications. Many members of the public have become increasingly sophisticated in the language of (primarily) medicine, and can talk meaningfully about the 'disorders' or 'illness' or 'conditions' that they believe afflict them or others around them. Such lay readers of this book also might want to know your *diagnosis*.

At our first meeting I had no interest in your diagnosis; that represented someone else's representation of whatever it was that ailed you. The diagnosis is an example of a *his*-story. At our first meeting my aim was to encounter *you*, not to recognize some features that were meaningful to the person who had referred you. This is not an antipsychiatric position, although it is often mistaken as such, especially by those who believe that one either *is* or *is not* in favour of the traditional approach to resolving problems of living by first identifying their common features – symptoms. At our first meeting I wanted to find out something of *who* you were. I needed to resolve some of my complete ignorance of Bobbie, the person. True, I knew something of who was Bobbie the *patient*. That information was contained in the referral letter. However, I viewed the process that might or might not unfold as a human undertaking, and for that I needed some human information. I needed to encounter the person. And so I filed the letter and got on with the engagement!

Behind this emphasis on the personal nature of the encounter lay an assumption that somewhere within this person lay the resources that might help to restore the balance, so to speak, of this temporarily unbalanced Bobbie[7]. These resources are not, of course, anything like the whole story of recovery, far less of overcoming, but involve their interface with the resources of others, not least the therapist. But this emphasis on resources marked another significant departure in my thinking from anyone else who would be interested to any great extent in your diagnosis. The diagnosis represents a primary classification of the human phenomenon (the patient) entirely from the perspective of what is wrong, deficient, malfunctioning, dysfunctional or plain disordered. A therapist who approaches a patient with bipolar disorder or agoraphobia may well focus, at some point, on the assets, strengths or human virtues of the patient. However, the simple act of assigning a diagnosis in the first place speaks a certain kind of truth about the unfolding therapeutic process. It marks[8] the beginning of the therapeutic process in a highly specific fashion. It declares the therapist's understanding of what the person has brought – or even what has brought the person – to therapy. Alternatively, I was interested to know your construction of events rather than to expose myself immediately to my sense, my understanding or my meanings.

As Thomas Szasz has eloquently summarized, the process of diagnosis is a process of *diminishment*, reducing the complexities of the human being and all that is represented *in* and *through* their 'problems of living' to a mere classification (Szasz, 1974a):

> [when] a psychiatrist [*sic*] classifies a newly admitted patient as a paranoid schizophrenic, he does exactly what Sartre described. The diagnostic label imparts a defective personal identity to the patient. It will henceforth identify him to others and will govern their conduct towards him, and his towards them. The psychiatric nosologist thus not only describes his patient's so-called illness, but also prescribes his future conduct.

Some have taken the view that Szasz, and indeed those like me who agree with the view stated above, reject the notion that people *suffer*. This is a crucial point and, as Szasz observed (Szasz, 1974b):

> I can only say that I consider the notion of mental illness a myth. Asserting this, I do not mean to deny the obvious fact that people may suffer from, and be disabled by, the difficulties that the task of coping with life presents to them. We must keep in mind, however, that mental illnesses

---

[7]This assumption was to find some support in one of your conclusions; that our relationship led to you gaining the capacity to trust others, yourself and the world. This appears to reflect Dostoevsky's intriguing suggestion that the biblical injunction to 'love thy neighbour as thyself' makes more sense if turned upside down – that is, one can love one's neighbour only if one loves oneself (cited by Watzlawick, 1983).

[8]Or perhaps more accurately, it *signals* a certain intention to view the person from a particular perspective. In so doing, it also signals a particular power relationship between therapist and patient.

are merely the names we give to certain strategies of living and their consequences.

Szasz represents a liberationist view of the human condition. He is interested in the *person* who expresses these various statements and tactics and manoeuvres as a way of living with his or her problems of living. He does not reserve this emphasis on the person, for people who become 'patients'. In a conversation a few years ago he told me about his return to Budapest, which he had left as a young man to emigrate to America. I asked him if he still felt like a Hungarian. 'No,' he answered, 'I do not feel like a Hungarian. But if you had asked me, "do I feel like an American?", I also would have said "No. I feel like *me!*".'

In approaching that first encounter with *you*, I was anxious to avoid casting you in the role of one type of patient or another. Indeed, I wanted to avoid casting you as any *type*[9], whether as function of your gender, your occupation, your race or whatever. I wanted to encounter the 'me' of which Tom Szasz was so rightly proud.

The therapist–patient relationship is predicated on a power game. Even where the therapist tries to meet the patient on something close to an equal footing, the patient is still disempowered – not just by the effects of the 'ailment/disorder', but also by being dependent (at least to some extent) on the outcome of the therapy. Although *sharing* the therapeutic relationship, *how* the therapist shares the experience is manifestly different from the patient.

By attributing a 'diagnosis' to someone's presentation (what the person brings to therapy), the therapist lays his or her cards on the table. In effect, the diagnosis betrays a certain view of the phenomena; it assigns a certain meaning. Although many therapists use the same diagnostic labels to express differing theoretical viewpoints, the use of the diagnosis infers that some kind of world view (or philosophical orientation) is being taken towards the phenomenon that is the patient. So a psychodynamic psychotherapist might interpret a 'chronic depression' as having 'a self-soothing function'[10], or the more biologically-minded therapist might assume that the phenomenon is 'related to reduced levels of the neurotransmitters serotonin and norepinephrine' (Feldman and Feldman, 1998). My world view is not in any way better than the views of other therapists or psychiatric professionals, but is only different. Indeed, I am willing to accept that my view of the inherent resourcefulness of the person-who-is-the-patient may be an entirely imaginary one, not grounded in any kind of empirically verifiable reality. However, having tried various other world views and theoretical assumptions on for

---

[9]Hence the common fear, at least among actors, of becoming *typecast*. All the other possible 'selves' that they might enact become occluded by the one role with which they have become associated.

[10]Or 'Even when depression is painful, it tends to reduce the impact of stimulation. Its presence usually suggests that some state of affairs has proven too much for the subject' (Eigen, 1993).

size, I have found them ill-fitting, where they were not downright uncomfortable. My assumptions as to your inherent resourcefulness were tailor-made for me. Indeed, they may be my first, rather than even a metaphorical second, skin. I suspect that the 'skins' worn by other therapists of different persuasions fit them just as snugly. It seems important that therapists feel comfortable in themselves; that they are *genuine*, in the way the Carl Rogers described (Rogers, 1995). If they try to fake it, I fear that they risk being found out[11].

The downside to genuineness is that if the therapist only has 'himself' to bring to the encounter, he may find that self wanting in the eyes of some patients. Honesty can, on occasions, be a doubtful policy.

Reflecting on the inter-relationship between yourself, the counsellor (C) and the analyst (A), you wrote first:

I was interested in what you had to say about 're-authorship'. Now there's a situation where the therapist has a lot of power and, speaking from experience, the patient feels powerless. Here is an example for you. During my last meeting with A she accused me of simply replacing C as I had found my way into the official system (psychoanalysis) relatively quickly after being dumped by him. At the time, and even now, I strongly disagreed with that view, but there didn't seem any point in actively disagreeing with the analyst. It didn't seem open to discussion. She had the power to decide things about my behaviour and reasoning, but I seemingly didn't have the power to alter her perceptions.

Then, turning to the counsellor, you noted:

About six months into counselling, the counsellor asked me if I would like to read his notes. After each session he would record what had happened and his thoughts. I was intrigued and apprehensive at the same time, but took the notes. It was there I read how he was irritated by all the things I did to 'control him'. He cited the relaxation exercises, the glass of water and my frequent decision to sit on the floor in a corner (where I felt more comfortable). I did these things to control my own feelings of disruption, not to control him. I still don't understand why such things can be seen as controlling him. Anyway, that was it. I stopped doing these things because by then I was hooked and wanted to please him, and couldn't cope with the thought of him getting angry with me over it.

The other thing I reacted to in the notes was his mention of T, who had been trying to encourage him to drop me because I was 'a bottomless

---

[11]Intellectually as opposed to emotionally, however, I have come to appreciate some of the problems of assuming that there can be any absolute truths about people, such as are assumed by medical or psychological theories. These belong in the masculine realm of the *proper*, which Cixous saw as expressing a possessive desire to territorialize, and therefore dominate, persons (Cixous, 1986).

*case'. This is important, because it had an effect on a subsequent
exchange with the analyst.*

*Having read this particular note, I stormed back to C and asked, who
was this guy T? He had stressed at the start how everything was confidential and he wouldn't share my secrets with anyone. Then suddenly T
appeared from nowhere. It turned out T was his supervisor. He explained
that all counsellors have a supervisor, adding 'He is your protection as
well as mine'. I must admit that these words have a pretty hollow ring
now. T became a real problem for me during therapy. I felt I was fighting
an unknown foe, someone that really didn't like me, and who wanted the
counsellor to dump me. However, 12 months before he did dump me C
assured me that he was 'his own man' and didn't always agree with
everything his supervisor said. Neither did he always follow his advice.
Maybe my life would have been a lot easier in the long run if he had.*

*Anyway, the point I am making here is that the analyst got very stroppy
with me when I made some comment about her telling her supervisor
about my weirdness. She had a rare moment of liveliness, and snapped
'I'm a consultant psychiatrist. I don't have a supervisor'. I can see now
that my comment was highly insulting to her, particularly as she was
being compared to someone (C) who she might consider to be a bogus
professional. But at the time I intended no insult, but had a genuine
concern to find out how far I could trust her. I was trying to develop my
appreciation of the system. I think this shows how important this re-
authorship thing is. I really wanted to make therapy with the analyst
work because I really wanted to get back to my old self and thought she
was my only chance to do that. Naturally it was going to be difficult for
me given all that had gone before. However, I think there were times we
could have made more sense of each other if she'd been more angled at
where I was coming from, rather than following a rigid technical
approach with an apparently rigid interpretation of my behaviour and
thoughts.*

These criticisms seem acceptable, although the reader might feel I would
say so, given that I appear to emerge from your appraisal unscathed, if
not heroic. As I said earlier, however, I don't think the point of therapy
(from the therapist's perspective) is to be successful; rather, it is to
provide the patient with conditions through which (s)he might become
whatever (s)he needs to become at that moment. The success of the
therapy lies in that moment. Like Kopp, I am confident that there are
some 'eternal truths' (Kopp, 1980) that might relate to therapy as well as
to patient and therapist. These may only be true for me and others like me
who come to appreciate them. Others may not be ready to embrace these
truths, or indeed for them they may never have the necessary 'ring' of
truth. Increasingly I believe that the search for the 'best' model of therapy
for any specific 'condition' is a vain and futile undertaking. It seems
obvious that the therapy – expressed by the whole presentation of the

therapist – must fit whatever it is that the 'person-of-the-patient' needs. And as you have illustrated throughout the previous chapters, those needs are shifting. If the therapist tries to hold fast to his own model of the world, he risks either losing the patient from his sight, or being pulled under as the patient sinks beneath the surface of her distress.

And in such a vein you wrote:

Often, when I looked at the analyst to gauge how I was being received, all I saw was the bowed head as she made copious notes. I had the unwarranted but very real feeling that everything I said was being taken down and would be used in evidence to label me a straitjacket-worthy case. I did not respond well to the psychoanalytical therapy. I experienced these sessions as oppressive silences, which I felt compelled to fill with I knew not what. Several times she told me that this was 'my hour' to talk about 'whatever I wanted'. However, I couldn't respond. I couldn't find a way into meaningnul soliloquy. Often I felt like shouting, 'If I knew what to do with myself, I wouldn't be here asking you for help!' I was looking for some magic trick that would make it all OK.

Rereading and reconnecting with your journals, I realize how often I too almost lost you from my sight. Often I too tended to lead you, when I should have been 'getting lost' in following you; checking to see what *you* appeared to need, as opposed to what I thought you needed. Thinking we know what the person has come to therapy in search of is perhaps one of the core psychotherapeutic conceits. At some point, however, I must have let myself go, allowing myself to discover what I have long believed to be the true wisdom of therapy – the therapist's intuitive appreciation of the patient's inherent resourcefulness; what might be called your 'homing instinct'.

Taking a horstory

The homing instinct can be illustrated best by retelling an apocryphal Milton Erickson tale[12]. One day when Erickson was out walking with a friend in the country, a mare galloped past them, riderless and without a saddle. The horse came to a stand in a nearby field. 'Must have got lost,' said Erickson, 'I'll take her back', as he mounted the mare, grasping the mane to steady himself. He turned the horse around and she set off back along the road. Erickson rode along, only gently pulling on the mane whenever the mare seemed to be straying into a field. After passing through several crossroads the mare turned into a small dirt road, and after a couple of miles they appeared at a farm. The farmer stood amazed

---

[12]I have no idea whether or not the story is true but, as my Irish forbears would say, why let the facts get in the way of a good story?

when he saw his horse. 'Gee, I thought she was gone for good. Where did you find her?' Erickson replied, 'oh, a few miles down the road.' 'But how did you know she was from here?', the surprised farmer asked. 'I didn't', answered Erickson, 'but *she* did'.

Does this sound too obvious? I guess the history of psychiatry, and to a lesser extent the history of psychotherapy, is a story about one group of people deciding (metaphorically) where people belong, and trying to help them get there. Often the process of getting people 'there' requires quite a lot of direction, since the person (patient) simply doesn't feel he or she belongs there. (In psychotherapy parlance, this is usually called *resistance).* The simple Ericksonian tale illustrates the value of following the patient, remembering that, like the horse, the patient needs to be treated carefully and respectfully, and will sometimes need the gentlest of nudges when she looks as if she is straying from her path. Of course, knowing that this is the right path is important, but, stretching the metaphor, often people discover a new 'destination' that feels more like home than the first one did. That kind of reconstruction often takes time, but can also occur dramatically as people realize the extent to which they had been stuck on the wrong road for so much of their lives.

Real therapy, and the problem of reality

Before I close, I should attempt to defend myself from the potential accusation of the reader that I am a fraudulent psychotherapist. Indeed, because I observed no specific therapeutic theory within the context of our work together, I might be accused of not really being a therapist at all[13]. We have not talked much about reality, since the whole business of therapy and illness – so imbued with metaphor – is not really about *reality (*paradoxical though that may sound). Rather, it is about some kinds of reality as opposed to others.

The great irony is that, as we begin a third millennium, at least to Western eyes we are rooted in a materialist conception of our 'selves' and our various worlds of experience. This appears, at least to me, to be a rejection of much of the progress in human understanding we have made over the last 1000 years. Instead of recognizing how we might have come to know, differently, some of the 'eternal truths', we still seek reassurance in a materialist conception of the universe. We still seek to deny not only God (like Nietszche) but also the problem of uncertainty, or the ineffability of the universe – human or otherwise.

---

[13]Although I have practised psychoanalytic, behavioural, humanistic, cognitive and family therapies, as well as hypnosis, on reflection the emphasis of my experience has been very much on *practice.* I have, through these various approaches, been rehearsing for the practice of being 'myself' in therapy: of developing my own gift of time (Barker, 1999).

I have betrayed some of my affiliations to an existentialist[14] reading of the psychotherapeutic encounter. This implies a specific 'reading' of reality which, perhaps, in this conclusion needs to be more formally articulated.

I have made reference at various points in previous chapters to Oriental thought, especially that of Taoist or Buddhist thinkers. Such reflections belong in the territory that Kopp so rightly, if ironically, defined as the Eternal Truths. The difference between the Oriental and Occidental minds of 2500 years ago might not be as wide as we now believe. Today, however, we are increasingly pushed to accept a materialist conception of the human universe, which might explain in part the emergence of the new age and its search for contact with the ineffable both within and outwith ourselves (Storm, 1994).

However, the rejection of a materialist interpretation of the human universe is not a new phenomenon. Over a hundred years ago Nietzsche rejected the religious tradition, and in so doing acknowledged that human experience was not, therefore, rational and meaningful in any fundamental sense. It was not part of any grand plan. Today we are encouraged to believe that the fundamental plan is approved either by our genetic code (Crick, 1994) or by the survivalist laws of neo-Darwinism (Dawkins, 1995).

Much of what you have described in your journals involves a search for understanding. This seems to me to wish to go beyond the simplistic explanations of our popular currency; that you feel threatened simply because contemporary events remind you of past events. However they are dressed up, many contemporary accounts of mental distress appear simplistic, reducing the person to the level of an animal who almost mechanically obeys a biopsychosocial rule, which ultimately may exist only in the minds of the theorist who formed the rule and subsequently published it for the widespread consumption of all who 'accepted' it. These laws assume that the limits of your human universe involve a cycle of interactions between the social world, your thoughts and the biological world that processes your thoughts, producing – as a by-product – your emotions.

I am inclined to assume, especially on reflection, that your various therapeutic struggles are characterized more by a search for yourself, which might ultimately be defined as spiritual, than simply by an attempt to remedy some troubling if disabling emotions. Much of what you appear to have achieved for yourself as a result of the therapeutic encounter involves awareness. You have become more aware of both the form and nature of your existence and, by implication, what it all might mean for you – its value. Perhaps the serenity – if I can use that term loosely – that

---

[14]By this term I mean all the thinkers who have sought to explore 'beyond reason' – Kierkegaard, Nietzsche, Sartre, Jaspers, Camus and Heidegger, as well as the Surrealists (in art) and the Theatre of the Absurd in literature, especially Samuel Beckett.

you have achieved has arisen from your awareness of something within yourself that might lie hidden within everyone. You may have encountered within yourself a 'silent partner' who has assisted you to appreciate the intelligibility, rather than the illogicality, of yourself and your reactions to life. The understandings you have finally acquired, unlike the simple remedies for your disabling anxiety that you learned to appreciate, may have helped you to clarify some of the meaning of your existence. Although to the materialist this may seem grandiose, to the Zen mind it is *knowing* that sometimes I am like this, and sometimes I am like that. The acquisition of such an understanding does not eliminate or cancel out the problems that once dogged your existence. Rather, you acquire a different relationship with them. Recall the famous Zen saying:

> Before enlightenment, mountains are mountains and water is water. When one gains an initiate's experience, this is denied, but when one gains enlightenment, everything is asserted again: mountains are mountains and water is water.

The difference lies not in the mountains and water, but in the nature of the relationship with the mountains and water.

We all struggle with such realizations day by day, whether we are in therapy or not and whether aware of it or not. Perhaps for all of us the goal is just such an awareness of our existence. It can become a full understanding, whilst being empty at the same time (Munitz, 1979):

> The Universe and men's [sic] lives, for all their meaningfulness and creative accomplishment, are set within the surrounding 'sea' of 'meaningless' and 'unintelligible' Existence. And the awareness of this fact is what comes to permeate and suffuse all one's experiences, whether happy or unhappy, momentous or trivial, filled with goodness or with horror, pain and evil. The awareness of Existence qualifies any and all of the experiences. The awareness of Existence is a 'silent partner' and 'unexpressed accompaniment', which makes possible the kind of serenity available to a human being without benefit of either religion or science. By means of it one learns to 'care and not to care' at the same time.

Signifying reality

At the end of her memoir *Girl Interrupted*, Susanna Kaysen recalled a day spent at the Frick Museum in New York. When she had first visited the museum she had been seventeen and thinking about her English teacher, who was with her, and whether or not he would kiss her. She was also wondering if she would fail to graduate from high school. These were her thoughts as she stopped in front of a painting by Vermeer, in which a girl looks out of the frame, ignoring her music teacher who stands stoutly at her side. The first time she saw the painting she felt a sense of warning, as if the girl had just drawn a breath in order to say 'Don't'. As she backed away from the painting, she felt that the girl was saying 'wait ... don't go!'

However, she did go and the teacher did kiss her and she did fail the year, and 'eventually' she wrote ' I went crazy.' *Girl Interrupted* (Kaysen, 1995a) is the story of Susanna Kaysen's compulsory hospitalization in Massachussetts in the late 1960s. The content for the book emerged only after she had written two other novels and gradually memories of her hospitalization began to emerge. *Girl Interrupted* is a powerful memoir, which reads like a quiet catharsis. There are no dramatic outpourings, but each page is filled with sad, often tragic descriptions of the failure of the hospital staff to understand not only *who* Susanna Kaysen was, but also what might have been ailing her.

The book ends with a second trip to the Frick, sixteen years later, accompanied by a new, rich boyfriend with whom she enjoyed a some-what volatile relationship. She has forgotten that she had ever been to the Frick, and when her boyfriend stomps off she is left alone in front of the Vermeer, within which the girl has changed. She is no longer urgent, but is sad. She appears to be looking out of the picture for someone who would see her. She reads the title of the picture – *Girl Interrupted at her Music* – and realizes (Kaysen, 1995b) how:

> my life had been, interrupted in the music of being seventeen, as her life had been, snatched and fixed on canvas: one moment made to stand still and to stand still for all the other moments, whatever they would be or might have been. What life can recover from that?

When her boyfriend returns to find her crying in the corridor, he chas-tizes her:

> Don't you see, she's trying to get out', she says pointing at the girl. 'All you ever think about is yourself. You don't understand anything about art'.

As she turns back to the painting, she notices something about the light in the three Vermeer paintings hanging before her. She realizes that the wall is made of light that is both credible but also unreal – a 'Vermeer light'. She realizes that:

> Light like this does not exist, but we wish that it did. We wish the sun could make us young and beautiful, we wish our clothes could glisten and ripple against our skins, most of all we wish that everyone we knew could be brightened simply by our looking at them

– as are the figures in the other two pictures. She concludes, however, that:

> The girl at her music sits in another sort of light, the fitful, overcast light of
> life, by which we see ourselves and others only imperfectly, and seldom.

This is one of the most elegant yet evocative summaries of the human
significance of mental distress that I have read. In a few lines the author
captures the disruptive effect of her breakdown on her life journey, which
left her in a kind of half-light that, on reflection, might cast a shadow
over most of us in differing kinds of ways.

The psychic pain of mental distress needs, perhaps, to be appreciated
for just what it *is*, before we come to consider what it might *do* to a life.
Psychic pain may leave people metaphorically in the shadows, partially
obscuring both who and what they are. But maybe we are all in a similar
kind of half-light, failing to really 'see' others for what they are, and
failing to appreciate ourselves by reflection.

Suzanna Kaysen sounds as if she is 'sadder but wiser' (Barker, 1992),
having developed some heartfelt wisdom about being both frail and
human – a wisdom that escapes her more headstrong boyfriend.
Certainly she evokes a compassion that was sorely lacking in those who
purported to 'care' for her. Sadder, wiser, and certainly not bitter.

I have no idea whether you have emerged from your own 'interruption'
sadder but wiser. I feel you have, but have no evidence (or at least none
that would pass muster in the empirical sense) with which to back that
up. Indeed, despite the current passion for collecting evidence to justify
the value we attach to health care – including psychotherapy – I am reluc-
tant even to ask you if my assumption is true. Perversely, I would rather
assume that you might be, since 'sadder but wiser' seems to be a very full
kind of human wisdom. If you have not found it, I hope that some day
you might. That would represent a dignified and deserved ending to this
chapter in your life story.

As we concluded this chapter, you drew an apposite parallel between
my 'intentional ignorance' of your emergence, and the tradition of teaching[15]:

*I am wondering if you are in effect saying that you don't want to know
how I have 'emerged'. Is this something to do with the reserve of teachers? (MacLaverty, 1998):*

'... you were a great teacher.'
'Nonsense, that was only the basic. Anyway, lessons are learned, not
taught.'

'No, a teacher is for a particular time. I needed to be taught those things
then. And in that way.'

---

[15]Perhaps you recognized the siginificance of the Latin root of 'doctor', meaning 'to teach'. Perhaps ,
after all, I was more concerned with fostering your education than in 'healing' you.

... She feels good about this. And suddenly she feels good about herself. Someday she will be better. Wellness was inside her, waiting on the edge of its seat. Like the Rose of Jericho. Ready to flower however long it has been dormant ...

This seems like a fitting point to begin to end this particular reflection, but I shall doubtless continue reflecting on your gentle challenge about teachers and teaching. Everything is true, for nothing is always true. Truth regularly makes room for other truths. However, like a mirror, truth and the reflecting process are endless and timeless, but we feel the need to mark them just the same. We fear, perhaps, that if we spend too long in front of the mirror it will capture us, or at least will steal the true essence of this moment – like the girl interrupted.

References

Barker, P. (1992) *Severe Depression: A Practitioner's Guide*. Chapman and Hall.

Barker, P. (1999). *The Talking Cures: An Introduction tot he Psychotherapies for Health Care Professionals*. NT Books.

Cixous, H. (1986). Sorties. In: *The Newly Born Woman* (H. Cixous and C. Clement, eds), pp. 82–96. Manchester University Press.

Clay, S. (1999). Madness and Reality. In: *From the Ashes of Experience: Reflections on Madness, Recovery and Growth* (P. Barker, P. Campbell and B. Davidson, eds), pp. 59–60. Whurr.

Cox, M. (ed.) (1992). Brian Cox interviewed by Rob Ferris. In: *Shakespeare Comes to Broadmoor: The Actors are come Hither. The Performance of Tragedy in a Secure Psychiatric Hospital* (M. Cox, ed.). Jessica Kingsley Publishers.

Crick, R. (1994). *The Astonishing Hypothesis*. Touchstone.

Dawkins, R. (2000). *The Blind Watchmaker*. Penguin.

Derrida, J. (1992). *Given Time: 1. Counterfeit Money*. University of Chicago Press.

Eigen, M. (1993). *The Psychotic Core*, p. 123. Jason Aronson Inc.

Facey, A. B. (1985). *A Fortunate Life*. Penguin.

Feldman, M. D. and Feldman, J. M. (1998). *Stranger than Fiction: When our Minds Betray Us*, p. 220. American Psychiatric Press.

Fox, N. (1999). *Beyond Health: Postmodernism and Embodiment*. Free Association Books.

Fromm Reichman, F. (1950). *Principles of University of Intensive Psychotherapy*. University of Chicago Press.

Hesse, H. (2000). *The Glass Bead Game*. Vintage.

Inglesby, E. (1992). Values and philosophy of nursing: the dynamic of change. In: *Nursing Care: The Challenge to Change* (M. Jolley and G. Brycsynska, eds), pp. 70–81. Edward Arnold.

Kaysen, S. (1995a). *Girl Interrupted*. Virago Press.

Kaysen, S. (1995b). *Girl Interrupted*, pp. 167–8. Virago Press.

Kopp, S. (1980). *If You meet the Buddha on the Road, Kill Him!* Sheldon Press.

MacLaverty, B. (1998). *Grace Notes*, p. 107. W. W. Norton.

Mauss, M. (1990). *The Gift: The Form and Reason for Exchange in Archaic Societies*. Routledge.

Moi, T. (1985). *Sexual Textual Politics*. Methuen.

Munitz, M. K. (1979). *The Ways of Philosophy*, p. 351. Collier Macmillan.

O'Hanlon W. H. and Beadle, S. (1997). *A Field Guide to Possibility Land*. BT Press.

Rogers, C. R. (1995). *On Becoming a Person*. Houghton Mifflin.

Shrock, R. A. (1982). Is health visiting a profession? *Health Visitor*, **55**, 104–6.

Storm, R. (1994). *Heaven on Earth*. Bloomsbury.

Sullivan, H. S. (1953). *The Interpersonal Theory of Psychiatry*. W. W. Norton.

Szasz, T. (1974a). *Ideology and Insanity: Essays on the Psychiatric Dehumanisation of Man*, pp. 198–199. Penguin.

Szasz, T. (1974b). *Ideology and Insanity: Essays on the Psychiatric Dehumanisation of Man*, p. 93. Penguin.

Watzlawick, P. (1983). *The Situation is Hopeless but not Serious*, p. 95. W. W. Norton.

Index

Accountability of therapist, 35
Action for change, 14, 83–5
Art therapy, 10
Attending appointments, 92–3
Awareness, 52–4, 64, 65, 92, 125,
   165–6
   of feelings, 95, 96
   noticing approach ('just being'),
   125–7, 144, 145

Beginning therapy, 14, 15, 22–3, 90,
   93–4, 96–7, 117–18
   finding a therapist, 23–9
Behaviour therapy, 9
Boundaries, 67

Change
   during therapy, 77–8, 85, 97,
   102–3, 108–9, 121–2, 147–8
   seeking therapy, 92
Client-centred therapy, 9
Coach model, 17, 62–3, 103, 119,
   122
Cognitive therapy, 9
Collaborative therapy, 16–17,
   121
Comfort, 131–2
Communication, 12, 28, 117, 118,
   119–20
   alternative forms, 59–60
   failure, 60–1, 115, 116–17
   finding a common language, 56–60

language of psychotherapy, 51–2,
   144
Conditioning therapy, 9
Consultation environment, 25, 29,
   32–3
Coping facilitation, 8
Coping methods, 41–2, 43, 48, 92, 93
'Core' human being, 95, 114
Counselling, 10–11, 58
   supervision, 162

Dependence, 11, 15, 48, 71
   starting therapy, 32
   unsuccessful therapeutic
   encounters, 24, 27, 28–9
Diagnosis, 158, 159, 160
Diary records, 15
Dignity, 133
Discovery, 40, 135, 136
Drama of human experience, 19–21,
   30

Education, 135–6
Empathy, 13, 57, 100, 115
Empowerment, 132
Enlightenment, 100, 137
Existential analysis, 9
Expert knowledge, 75
Exploration of patient's experience,
   36, 40–1, 44, 46, 49, 153–4
   language for communication,
   59–62, 64

therapist's role, 75–6
  timing, 43, 142
Faith in therapeutic system, 13
Family therapy, 9
Fear of failure, 137, 139
Felt knowledge, 135, 136, 149
Focus of therapeutic endeavour, 38,
    39, 43, 86–7
Friendship, 98

Genuineness, 13, 162
Goals of therapy, 6, 7, 33, 48, 49,
    57–8, 63
  continuous learning, 86
  patient's expectations, 69
  self-discovery, 114
Good authority, 11–12
Group analysis, 9
Growth, 89–90, 94, 108, 110, 136–7,
    139, 140
Guidance, 8
Guide model, 62, 63
Guilt feelings, 99

Healing, 1, 4
Hearing, 57, 136, 155
Helpful interventions, 23
Holistic approaches, 5, 6
Homework assignments, 15–16, 83–4,
    141, 143, 145
Human nature, 95, 114
Humanistic approaches, 5, 6, 95,
    114
Hypnosis, 10

Impermanence of experience, 44–5
Information uptake, 144
Inner voice of patient, 2, 3
Inner wisdom, 124, 125
Insight, 65
Interdependent needs in therapy,
    70–1, 85–7

Language, 51–2
  power of words, 54, 55–6, 64–5
  of psychotherapy, 51–2, 144

Leap of faith, 101, 112–15, 120–1,
    122, 124, 125, 132, 133
Learning, 86, 135–6
Listening, 57, 155
Loss, 42, 43, 101, 102

Madness, 145–6
Marital therapy, 9
Meditation in life, 125–7, 144, 145
Mental distress of patient, 4, 159–60,
    168
  emotional meaning, 100–2
Music, 60

Needs of patient, 97, 164–5
Needs of therapist, 70, 71, 85, 136
Non-directive approach, 54–5, 59,
    118, 119, 163
Normal life committments, 31–2
Noticing (meditation in life), 125–7,
    144, 145

Outcome assessment, 150–3, 169

Patient status, 20
Patient's expectations, 69, 73, 74
Peace of mind, 131
Person–centred approach, 95
Personal agency, 132–3
Philosophic therapy, 9
Physical activity, 43
Play therapy, 10
Post-traumatic stress disorder, 38, 99
Power differential/dynamic in therapy,
    11, 26, 27, 31, 73, 153, 156–7,
    160, 161
Practical wisdom, 100
Problems of patient, 2, 5, 38–9, 47,
    93, 158–59
  assessment for referral, 113
  family/spouse distress, 76
  mental distress, 4
  resolution, 130
  stages of therapeutic process, 14
Professional distance, 67
Progress, 47–8, 129

Psychiatric labels, 50–1, 132–3, 144, 145–6
Psychoanalysis, 6–8
Psychoanalytic (psychodynamic) psychotherapy, 7–8, 9
  method, 58, 68, 74, 75
Psychodrama, 9
Psychotherapy
  aims *see* Goals of therapy
  definitions, 1, 4–5
  functions, 8–10
  historical development, 4–6
  methods, 5

Rational-emotive therapy, 9
Re-authoring/reframing, 104, 105–8, 153–4
Re-educative psychotherapy, 9
Reality
  acceptance, 137–8
  Eastern philosophic concepts, 2–3, 165, 166
  relationship to words ('construction' in therapeutic conversation), 63–4, 77, 78
  therapist's world view, 55, 164, 165
Reassurance, 8, 94, 113
Reconstructive psychotherapy, 9–10
Recovery process, 129–30, 141, 147, 158–9
Reflection, 45, 46, 83
Reflective process, 97, 100, 115
Restoration of basic trust, 13, 153
Restoration of morale, 12
Risk taking, 112, 121, 141
Role of therapist, 75–6

'Safe space', 12–13, 48
Seeking therapy, 23–9, 37–8, 92, 93, 103, 112–13
Self
  change over time, 37
  reconstruction during therapy, 87
  therapeutic use, 35
Self-awareness, 92
  of therapist, 35–6

Self-concept, 143
Self-consciousness, 109
Self-discovery, 114
Self-esteem enhancement, 8
Self-healing, 70, 80, 95, 114
  liberating patient's potential, 119, 128
Social approval, 142–3
Socratic dialogue, 97
Soul-work, 31
Supportive psychotherapy, 8–9

Talking cure, 4, 58
Termination stage of therapy, 14–15, 103–5, 122, 147, 148, 150–1
Termination of therapy, 24, 29, 73
Therapeutic alliance, 51, 67
Therapeutic methods, 58–9, 87
Therapeutic process, 14–15
  action for change, 14
  beginning, 14
  termination, 14–15
  understanding problem, 14
Therapist-patient relationship, 5, 11, 13
  co-operative therapy, 16–17, 121
  communication, 12, 56–60
  consultation environment, 25, 29, 32–3
  dependence, 48
  development of relationship, 36–8, 44, 62–3, 72–4, 76–87
  engagement, 30–1, 34, 74–6, 155
  interdependent needs, 70–1, 85–7
  language of psychotherapy, 51–2, 144
  personal element, 68, 74–5, 76
  power dynamic, 11, 26, 27, 31, 73, 153, 156–7, 160, 161
  risk taking, 112, 121
  starting therapy, 32, 44
  therapist's knowledge, 21, 64, 75
  trust, 114, 115–16, 120, 122, 123, 152
  unsuccessful encounters, 24–8, 30, 72–3, 96, 118, 154, 161–2, 163

Therapist's attributes, 11–13
    asking good questions, 56, 77
    choice of therapeutic approach, 58, 87
    communication skills, 12
    curiosity about patient's world, 76–7
    encouragement, 12
    good authority, 11–12
    provision of direction, 12
    provision of 'safe space', 12–13
Therapist's knowledge, 21, 64, 75
Trance, 93
Transactional analysis, 9
Trust, 114, 115–16, 120, 122, 123, 152

Uncertainty, 39, 68–9, 108, 110, 124, 130, 164
Unconditional positive regard, 13
Unhelpful thoughts, 144
Unpredictability, 68

Validation as goal of therapy, 63

Warmth, 13, 115
Wholeness as goal of therapy, 33
Work, 125, 126
Work of therapy, 30–1, 53, 79, 80, 81, 128–9, 156
    asking good questions, 56, 77
World views, 55, 142, 160